Save the Bones

Shannon O'Donnell

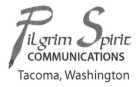

Tacoma, Washington

Additional material Copyright © 2016 by Shannon O'Donnell
Original Copyright © 2013 by Shannon O'Donnell
All Rights Reserved.

ISBN: 978-0-9826160-4-8

Cover Design: Alan Dubinsky
Additional Graphics: Kim Rivard, Graphic Point Design
Book Design: Judith Jones, Pilgrim Spirit Communications

Published in the United States of America by
Pilgrim Spirit Communications, Tacoma, Washington

No part of this book may be reproduced in any form without written permission of the author.

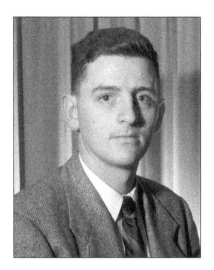

For Robert Austin O'Donnell

The father I don't remember

The husband my mother cannot forget

Contents

Are We There Yet?..1

Be Here Now 73

Now Where Are We? 113

After Stories 148

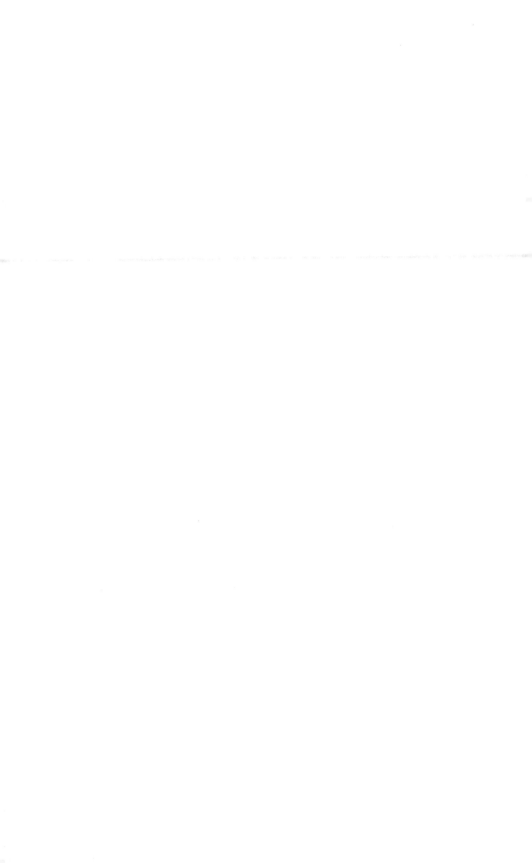

Singing in the ER

It's early January 2005. Mom and I are in St. Peter's Hospital in Olympia, in the emergency room. Mom fell shortly after lunch and we're here to get x-rays and find out if there's been any damage. She broke her hip last fall and may have compressed the pins that are holding her together now. Once she has a blanket, she dozes. Her feet are covered with bright red snowman socks. She takes pride in her socks. She has a collection to rival any I've ever seen.

"Where are we?" she asks, waking for a bit.

"At the hospital. Waiting for x-rays."

"Who pushed me?"

This is a familiar question. "No one pushed you. You fell."

"So what are we waiting for?"

"We're waiting for the bone doctor to tell us about the x-ray."

"Bone doctor? You're kidding me. Bone doctor?" And then she breaks into song, "Save the bones for Henry Jones, 'cause Henry don't eat no meat!" She laughs. "Where are we?"

I'm still laughing over the song but I tell her again that we're at the hospital, that she fell, that we're waiting for the bone doctor.

A week later, I'll be driving into the parking lot at work and that song will be on a local jazz station on the radio. "Save the bones for Henry Jones!" Nat King Cole and Johnny Mercer came out with this song in 1947, when Mom was in high school. Of all the songs she sang when we were kids, this is not one of them, but it is so like her. I don't get out of the car until I hear the whole thing.

Save the Bones for Henry Jones

(Danny Barker / Michael Goldsen [aka Vernon Lee] / Henry Jones)

We're gonna have a supper
We'll eat some food that's rare
And at the head of the table
We'll place brother Henry's chair
Invite all the local big dogs
We'll laugh and talk and eat
But we'll save the bones for Henry Jones
'Cause Henry don't eat no meat

Copyright 1947 Criterion Music Co.

Part I:
Are We There Yet?

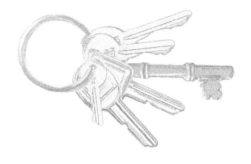

Introduction

I read the checklists in the newspapers and magazines. They promise to let me know how I can prevent Alzheimer's. You know the list: do the crosswords, read a lot, stay active, take a class. Every time I look at a list, I get angry. It doesn't work. Or it didn't, not for my mom.

My mother was never a typical woman. As long as I've known her, Marie Margaret Ultsch O'Donnell Cain has been fascinated by the world. For decades, she had subscriptions to, and read, three newspapers a day. When I was young, still living at home, the *Santa Maria Times*, the *Santa Barbara News-Press*, and the *San Francisco Chronicle* all made an appearance and were devoured. Magazines, especially ones featuring travel, food and gardening, found their way to side tables, book cases, and the shelf in her headboard. She was forever tearing out and trying some new recipe, suggesting a day trip to an interesting site, finding out a new bit of history to enhance yet another excursion to a museum. She supported the local drama departments at the high school and junior college with season tickets. She found ways to get us tickets to silent film festivals.

She traveled. She loved San Francisco when she lived there and one time, the two of us stopped at every single mission between Santa Barbara and San Francisco. There is one every seventeen miles. She knew that. The trip took us all day and into the night, but we saw every mission. In later years, she went to Ireland, France, and Japan.

I'd get great letters from her, usually several pages front and back, on stationery that no one else seemed to use anymore. The envelope would be crammed with clips from newspapers and magazines. There were notes written in the margins.

All of that and still she got Alzheimer's. It wasn't fair. It still isn't. The woman who loved politics and government doings and didn't hesitate to make her opinions known got the disease that robbed her of speech, stole her memories, and devastated the landscape that was her life. And yet.

Life with my mother didn't go from wonderful to awful in one fell swoop. It took time and "awful" isn't the right word for it anyway. What the lists never tell you, what the articles rarely say, is that some of this Alzheimer's stuff is damn funny. Maybe you have to have a certain warped sense of humor. Maybe you need a crown on your head and a name change to Cleopatra, Queen of Denial. Maybe you just need to know my mom.

I wrote this book because I got tired of the lists that don't bring my mother back, that tell me somehow she failed to protect herself from this disease, to care for herself well enough to avoid the mess. I wrote this book because I tell my friends some of these stories when they ask how my mom is doing. Their laughter teaches me: maybe there's something that hasn't yet been said about Alzheimer's. So I'm going to say it. "Funny" may not be on your list of words to describe the Memory Robber, but it's part of my experience.

I also wrote this book because I discovered that writing was one way I could deal with the confusion on all sides. I am baffled to be a caretaker of sorts and regularly have to work through what I'm supposed to be doing. Inevitably, I come to a point where I can only do what I do. Our lives have much in common with other people in similar circumstances, but no one plan works for everyone.

What I have known over the past dozen years is not the same for any other family. We come to this strange place from all different life circumstances and previous challenges. Humor is one way I stay sane; maybe that's why I've been able to find the fun in the interactions with my mother. Not that those interactions are always fun. Sometimes they were, and are, darned exasperating. Hindsight, compassion, and time add depth to the picture.

This is one story in the flood of many. Welcome in. May you find some echo of your own story here. I promise: no lists.

Your Mother Called

The most valuable lesson I've learned about family is this: we are each entitled to our separate relationships with our parents and with our siblings. For many years, a conversation between any two of us included the words, "Your mother called." Never mind that she is our mother; in moments of crisis or stress, she is *your* mother.

It doesn't matter that our family came out two girls, four boys, in that order. Nor that the brothers were most often referred to as The Boys, two words that described the male crowd that included other boys in the neighborhood, intent on one high-powered adventure after another. Long into their adult years, "The Boys" is still useful shorthand.

The divisions were sharp when we were kids, marked mostly in my imagination by this wish: Maybe when we're adults we'll be friends. Today, with all of us in our fifties, we live on the West Coast, in three different states, a physical and emotional distance from each other.

This book is about our mother and Alzheimer's. More specifically, it is about my experience with Mom and Alzheimer's. We six siblings have our individual moments which overlap only rarely. I write from the middle of my own life and I haven't asked my siblings to write about theirs. That is a deliberate choice, born of our peculiar history and dynamics. Every family has its own.

We're driving in Mom's Cadillac. She runs a stop sign and we're almost hit by another car. I scream.

She yells, "I don't need you screaming in the car!"

"I don't need to be dead!"

Is This the Beginning?

It's January of 2002. My sister Erin and I plan a trip to Santa Barbara. It's been a while since we've seen Mom and we have a plan. It's been harder for Mom to keep in touch with everyone lately, so we have found an email machine for her. Nothing as fancy as a computer, just a machine that she can use to send and receive emails. Her hearing has gotten so bad that she is exasperated with phone calls. This seems like an easy solution. I make a list of instructions to take her through the process.

Mom's delighted to hear we're coming, thrilled to see us, takes us out to dinner. We tell her we're planning to stay a few days and to take her out shopping and sightseeing. We explain about the email machine. She doesn't get it, can't quite picture what we mean. She has been retired for almost ten years and she got out before computers were the big deal in any office. But we tell her we'll show her and teach her how to use it, that it will be fun for the grandkids to have a way to keep in touch. She likes the sound of that.

We call our brother Theo who lives an hour away and invite him to bring his girls down for a visit. We wait to tell Mom that he's coming until an hour beforehand, hoping to avoid any drawn out questioning. But Mom goes into a rant about how pissed she is at him. We don't understand why. Finally we get her to focus on the kids. She behaves herself during the visit, but it clearly wears her out.

Another night, we take her to dinner. She says she's starving, that she hasn't eaten since breakfast. But she had pizza, and a banana she found on the walkway, and dinner at the retirement home. I lose count of the times I answer, "What time does your plane leave?"

Ninety minutes with her and I'm zonked. We'll go over all this again in the morning, run her through another lesson on the email machine, and she should be okay.

Mom never uses the machine, never mentions it again. She complains it has been years since any of her kids visited. "And why are you calling me now? It's lunch time and they are waiting for me."

Scenes with My Mother

PHONE CALL (late night)

MARIE: I've decided to move. They don't want me here anymore.

SHANNON: Mom? Hello? What's going on?

MARIE: I'm being evicted.

SHANNON: Where are you moving to?

MARIE: Why should I move?

SHANNON: You said they're evicting you.

MARIE: Evicting me! What did I ever do that they'd evict me? I'll sue!

SHANNON: Mom, what's going on? It's late. Can we talk about this tomorrow?

MARIE: Don't call me if it's too late for you to talk.

SHANNON: I didn't call. You called—

MARIE: Don't talk to me like that. *(hangs up)*

PHONE CALL #2 (later that night)

SHANNON: Mom's being evicted.

GEOFF: What? Says who?

SHANNON: She does. She says she got a letter from management and she has to move.

GEOFF: *(laughs)*

SHANNON: She says other people are being evicted. That management doesn't like their politics.

GEOFF: I wrote her a letter. Gave her some good reasons why she should think about moving. Jacqui and I moved from Santa Barbara. She'll be closer to more family there in Washington. There's no one near her now.

SHANNON: *You* wrote her a letter?

Another night, another late phone call:

SHANNON: Let's talk about moving Mom from Santa Barbara to Tacoma.

GEOFF: It won't be pretty.

SHANNON: No kidding.

Storm on the Horizon

Mom lived in Santa Barbara for several years after she retired. It was the nearest Big City when we were all growing up. With its mission, art galleries, local politics, and a university, there was much to see and do. I heard about it in phone calls and letters Geoff and Jacqui, my brother and sister-in-law, were right there. They helped Mom with the shopping and banking, ran interference with legal things. They were the ones who helped her with the search for a retirement home and finally managed that change from independent apartment living.

Mom had an accident in a parking lot. She ran the car onto a median. She got out of the car, wandered away, and then didn't remember the accident or where her car was. She was hysterical. Geoff took the brunt of it when he told her it was time to give up driving. "Do we wait for you to kill someone with this car before we take the keys away?" For that, he became the Evil One.

Other things happened, most notably, meltdowns in public when she got frustrated and confused. What my sister and I saw on our brief visits was happening more consistently then we knew. The paranoia that often comes with Alzheimer's flashed even then. Mom was convinced that Geoff wanted to lock her away in a hospital.

Moving to a retirement home worked, for a while. There were activities and outside trips. But when Mom started signing up for everything and then not showing up, when she got into raging fights with other residents or the staff, then it was time to start thinking about doing something else. We started to consider assisted living. We all needed to shift.

Moving from Santa Barbara

May 2003. At the airport in Santa Barbara. Mom hasn't flown anywhere in a while. Members of the National Guard stand with rifles near the doors to the airport as we approach the security checkpoint.

SECURITY: Take off your shoes.

MARIE: Sweater? I'm not wearing a sweater.

SHANNON: Your shoes, Mom. Take off your shoes.

MARIE: Why?

SECURITY: It's required. Take off your shoes.

MARIE: I don't know why you want my shoes. *(takes them off)* Maybe my feet stink. Will that make you happy?

SECURITY: Go through the security gate. *(She ignores him)* Ma'am!

MARIE: What?

SHANNON: This way, Mom. Through the gate.

SECURITY: *(to Marie)* You have been randomly selected for a more thorough security check. Step this way please.

MARIE: *(to Shannon)* What is he flapping his gums about?

SHANNON: He wants to check you.

MARIE: Give me chicken?

SHANNON: *(enunciating)* To check you. *(guides Marie to station)*

SECURITY: *(to Shannon)* You can't be here.

SHANNON: She's deaf. She has Alzheimer's. And she hasn't heard a word you've said yet.

SECURITY: You can't be here. *(Shannon turns away)*

MARIE: Where are you going? Come back here! Don't leave me with this clown!

(SECURITY wands her.) Get away from me with that thing. *(She takes a swing at him.)*

SHANNON: Put your shoes on, Mom. Let's go. It's time for the plane.

Finally, we get past security, get her shoes back on—and my brother and his three kids show up. We go outside to say goodbye to them. When we come back in, SECURITY motions to Mom.

SECURITY: You've been selected for an extra security check. Please step over to the side.

MARIE: What?

SECURITY: Take off your shoes.

MARIE: Cheese? What cheese?

SHANNON: Can't you search me instead? She's already been through this once.

SECURITY: Ma'am, take off your shoes. Turn around.

Somehow we get on the plane without threatening national security and without anyone filing charges.

Interview

The plan is to get Mom into assisted living. There's just an interview and a test.

INTERVIEWER: Good morning, Marie. How nice to meet you.

MARIE: *(hasn't heard Interviewer)* Hello. I'm Marie Cain. Have you met my daughter?

INTERVIEWER: I'm going to ask you some questions. Is that okay?

MARIE: Fine with me.

INTERVIEWER: When is your birthday?

MARIE: *(puzzled)* I think in August. At least that's when we celebrate it. I'm getting too old for birthdays. Shannon's birthday is in August too. So is Theo's. He's one of my sons. I have four sons. Two daughters. We have lots of birthdays in August.

INTERVIEWER: That's great. Now, what year is it?

MARIE: Two thousand....something. I haven't worried about the date since I retired.

INTERVIEWER: Who is the president?

MARIE: That damn Bushie. *(to Shannon)* I can't stand that man. What were people thinking?

INTERVIEWER: *(tries not to laugh)* Here's something a little harder. Can you spell WORLD backward?

MARIE: World?

INTERVIEWER: Yes, can you spell it backward?

MARIE: T-I. *(she laughs, the Interviewer is uncertain, then gets the joke)*

INTERVIEWER: I like your sense of humor. We'd like you to spend the night with us. Try out the dining room and—

MARIE: I'm a vegetarian.

INTERVIEWER: Really?

SHANNON: True—for a very long time. Can your staff handle that? When I called—

INTERVIEWER: I'm sure we could make some arrangements. How unusual.

SHANNON: She's always been ahead of her time.

INTERVIEWER: Let me show you to our guest room. Your apartment will be like this one. This will give you a chance to get to know the place.

MARIE: Pretty bland in here.

SHANNON: Mom! It's just for a day or two. See how you like it. Your place will be different.

INTERVIEWER: Here are your keys. This one is for the door, the other for the mailbox. I'll see you at dinner. *(Marie inspects the room, then the keys)*

MARIE: I don't understand these keys. I can't tell them apart. How am I going to remember?

SHANNON: Little one is the mailbox.

MARIE: I don't understand.

We had such hopes. But that assisted living place didn't work out. According to Mom, she flunked the test. They also flunked— not being able to provide what she needs for activities and her vegetarian diet. There will be phone calls and visits to more facilities. Mom is waiting for the moving truck to arrive with her things from California. She needs familiar things around her. It's strange having her so close, but it will be good in the long run.

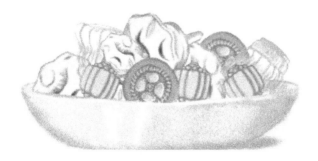

Finding Friends

My mother has always been a social woman with a huge variety of friends and acquaintances. She has always been independent and thinks nothing of planning a visit to a museum or a distant city on her own. Half the fun of knowing her has been to hear of the adventures she has created in new places.

Then she moved from a retirement home in Santa Barbara with hopes of joining a retirement community in Tacoma. In fact, it was the same place her father had lived the last years of his life. He had his own apartment and could come and go as he pleased. Even when he stopped driving, at 91, he still went out in the van with friends for shopping and lunch. When he died at 93, he was on a trip to Reno with some of those same friends.

Mom visited him a number of times there, staying in a visitor's apartment, meeting the residents, and admiring the selection of activities available both inside and out in the city. When she decided to move north, it was Grandpa's place she planned on. She didn't get her wish.

As we prepared for the move, it became clear that she needed a little more help: some supervision with her medications, maybe a room without a stove so she could avoid mishaps, someplace that could support her if her health declined. Fortunately, the retirement home had an assisted living section, so we checked into that. Her acceptance would hinge on a check-up with a doctor and a two-day trial stay.

The doctor visit went reasonably well. The two-day stay did not. In the end, Mom needed more specific care than assisted living provided. We went looking for Alzheimer's care facilities and that's how we ended up in Olympia at a wonderful place where the residents were respected and cared for with dignity. Mom thought her room was too small, that her king-sized bed would never fit (but it wasn't coming from California anyway, so I didn't worry about that much), that her vegetarian ways would be a problem. We got her moved in, ordered a phone, made sure she had subscriptions to her favorite newspapers, and waited for things to settle down. It would take a while for her to feel at home, so much had changed for her, there had been so much upset in her routine.

I was able to see her often. Her place in Olympia was halfway between my home in Tacoma and my work further west. I stopped in a couple of times a week. We went shopping at the Goodwill for knick-knacks and at clothing stores for new things. We tried out all sorts of restaurants. It was almost like the days when I used to visit her in California when we were both much younger.

In the fall of that year, I called a local parish to see if they might have volunteers who'd visit Mom. She found the other residents a challenge, to put it nicely. They were "boring, uninteresting, couldn't (or wouldn't) read a newspaper if their lives depended on it." Clearly she needed more than me to provide entertainment. I had a good chat with the volunteer coordinator who promised to visit Mom, interview her, and match her up with someone suitable. I checked that task off my list.

A few days later, Charlie called me back. "Is your mother always that mean?" he wanted to know. Mean? MY mom? I rolled my eyes and asked him to explain. He'd gone to see Mom the day before, in the morning, when she was most likely to be alert and engaged. Even though I'd told her about his visit, she had a difficult time understanding why he was there and what his intentions were. When it was finally clear, she erupted. She was insulted. She had no need of his services. And get the hell out. Now!

"I'm sorry," I said. This was not the first or the last time I would have to apologize for her. "I know she can be difficult sometimes." Charlie didn't think it would be a good fit for any of his team of volunteers. I thanked him and hung up.

The next day, I stopped to see Mom, intending to take her out to dinner. She refused to talk to me. She was spitting furious. "How dare you! You think I can't make friends on my own so you try to buy them for me?" Nothing would appease her. I left.

The next weekend, she called to see if we were going out to dinner when I left work on Sunday. She'd forgotten all about Charlie's visit. I never did try to buy her friends again.

Baby Book

There is a baby book somewhere
    notes my mother made
    the first time
    I smiled
    and rolled over
    sat up alone.
A blonde curl clipped from
    the first haircut
A ribbon from my baptism dress
    and wisdom from a toddler.

The baby book lived for a time
    in a stack
    of baby books
    that got thinner
    by the child.
By the time the sixth was born,
    there was a notation
    Mom got home in time
    for Christmas
    but not much else to mark
    his birth.
By #6, the newness is ordinary.

I have a book now
filled with wisdom
from my mother:
    "I don't know where I am.
    Where have I gone?"

Dinner will be here in half an hour.
    "Half an hour!
    I'll be dead by then!"

"I'm waiting for someone
    to run through the halls
    naked.
    Do you think I could plant
    the idea?
Stand back and watch!"

And then the notes shift
    things Mom needs to know:
You are in the hospital.
    Your hip is broken.
        Stay in bed.

Then there are gaps
    nothing unique any more.

Two books
    the beginning of a life
    the fading of another.

Dinner Time

October 2003

Daylight Savings Time ended last night and the sun is at an unfamiliar angle. It is time for dinner, but it seems like mid-afternoon. No matter. If it is five o'clock, we will eat!

The dining room is a bright clean place with seating for thirty people, if that many decide to come to dinner. Some of the tables are set for one or two, others for six. The tablecloths are deep green plastic with dark flowers on them. The chairs look comfortable. The menu is handwritten on a chalkboard on the wall. Tonight's main dish is egg salad sandwiches, accompanied by chicken noodle soup. I cannot resist wondering which will come first.

The residents come in, most looking slightly disoriented because the sun doesn't seem to be in the right place. "Are you sure it's time for dinner?" one tiny woman asks a young worker.

"Yes, it is, Myrna. Sit right on down." The worker, Connie, is cheerful. She takes Myrna's wrist and leads her to her place at a table set for six. Myrna hesitates when she reaches her chair, but with a bit of coaxing, she sits down. She straightens her silverware. Connie brings her a cup of tea and promises dinner will arrive shortly.

Adam, a slender older man, stands at the door of the dining room. His body is bent in half, supported by a walker. Gravity seems to be getting the best of him. Charlie, young with a substantial mustache, stands behind him, his palm resting on Adam's back, gently guiding him into the room. Adam resists and tries to move his walker down the hall. Charlie is persistent and gets Adam to his place at a table. Adam stands with his hands on the table while Charlie slides the chair into place. Then Adam must be convinced that he can sit down. Eventually, he does. Five minutes later, gravity overcomes him and Adam is face down on the table, his eyes focused on the tablecloth.

"The Girls" arrive in a group. There are five of them, all dressed up a bit, as if going out to dinner has always been an occasion. One carries a doll with her and rocks it. Another put on rouge for the evening. It is very red and applied slightly too high on her cheek bones. The ladies settle into their places and adjust their napkins. Nance polishes her silverware. "You just can't be too sure," she explains, but no one listens. The conversation ebbs and flows at their table. Their voices rise in heated debate. A worker approaches and listens, finally saying, "You all live here now. You're going to have to work it out."

"Says who?" asks the woman with the doll.

Dinner is served. My companion at the table inspects her plate. Her egg salad sandwich is served with a slice of tomato on it. She points this out and asks if the tomato is one of the perks of being a vegetarian. She gets cottage cheese instead of chicken noodle soup.

At another table Teresa, with her well-sculpted eyebrows and too-black hair, sits with Joan. Joan is new and in a wheelchair. Teresa wears a crisp white outfit and a bright pink scarf. Joan says something to her and Teresa responds, "I can't hear a thing you're saying. And I probably don't want to."

Joan looks puzzled. She tries again. "I couldn't stand to be like some of the people here. I'd shoot myself."

Teresa waves a hand at her. "Don't do that. Makes too big a mess." Joan shrinks into her wheelchair.

Sam and Leslie sit at a table next to the window. Leslie keeps her eyes closed through the meal. Her hand is frozen, halfway to her mouth, as if she has forgotten the path to get food from her plate to her mouth. Every now and then, Sam gets up, guides her hand, and tells her to take a bite and chew. Leslie wears a purple crash helmet. Dinner can be dangerous.

Forty minutes later, Teresa is still at her table, but Joan has moved on. Most of The Girls have gone as well. Only Jackie stays behind. Teresa looks at her, twists her mouth and points her finger at Jackie. "You're crazy," she proclaims.

Jackie protests. "You don't know my doctor!"

"I don't need to know your doctor. I know you and you're crazy."

Jackie is furious. She throws her napkin but it only sails to the floor. She struggles to her feet. If she could, she would stomp out of the room. She settles for a loud sniff.

Teresa takes another sip of her coffee. "Bitches. All of them."

Mom: Is this doctor going to look inside my mouth?

Me: No, not this time.

Mom: Then I won't brush my teeth.

At the Eye Doctor

September 2004

We saw the eye doctor today. I'm getting used to the comedy routine that we must present. In order to get Mom from the waiting room to the exam room, the receptionist calls her name, I poke her on the arm and point to the open door. Mom looks at me and says, "What?" I stand, help her up and then walk her toward the exam room. "Where are we going?"

"To get your eyes examined."

"There's nothing wrong with my mind," she protests. "I'm perfectly fine."

"I know you are. But this doctor wants to check your eyes." I point at my eyes and blink at her.

"Oh. I can do that," she decides. She goes into the exam room and sits in the chair. The doctor greets her and introduces himself.

"I'm Marie. Who are you?" asks Mom. The doctor introduces himself again. Mom looks at him. "I wear two hearing aids, for God's sake. Speak up!" She glares at me and snaps, "Do they teach everyone to mumble in medical school?"

"Sorry, she gets like this sometimes." Apologizing for my mother is wearing thin but it must be done. The optometrist assures me he sees plenty of patients who are like my mother. "She does have a hard time hearing," I explain. "My voice is one that she can hear fairly consistently."

And so the exam begins. The doctor asks questions, I repeat the question to Mom, Mom answers. Every few minutes she wonders what he is looking for inside her head.

In the end, her current prescription is fine. She should continue the eye drops for glaucoma. It was nice to meet you.

"Is that it? You shine lights in my eyes and ask questions and you've just now figured out I'm fine?" The doctor nods. He learns quickly.

"Get me out of here." I do.

No Filters

It's a place with no filters, no "I shouldn't say that out loud" censors. All the things I ever wished I could say, that I sometimes mumble out of the corner of my mouth, or scrawl on paper for a friend to read, all those things the people at the Alzheimer's care facility say. It is not freedom for them. It is simply how they are.

My mother is wickedly funny when she's in the mood. She may greet someone pleasantly, but if the other person doesn't respond, or, more likely, when Mom doesn't hear the response, as soon as the person turns away, Mom makes a face or sticks out her tongue or puts her hands to her ears and waggles them.

She says the women are boring, that they've led dull lives, "probably stayed home and baked cookies." The men she can talk to about work, but there are few of them and most have become silent. Simon, with his bright round eyes, was the head of a county health department in another state. He smiles, pushes his walker filled with National Geographics and a calendar stuck on November 2002, and never says a word.

Mom gets confused about time these days. We came back from Easter dinner and she was ready for another meal. She thought it was lunch time. She didn't remember the eggplant parmesan she'd finished half an hour before.

I wonder what she'll think when she opens her purse and discovers the check she started to write to me. She paid for dinner with her credit card and, for once, didn't tell me that she'd just gotten it in the mail a few weeks ago.

We have settled into a routine of sorts. She is busy at the care facility, though she's sleeping more during the day. I stop to see her and go to dinner at least once a week. She likes the outings but is glad to be home again.

Much like before, when she was living in Santa Barbara and Erin and I would visit, I am the upset in her routine, so we keep the interruptions at a minimum. It is not an easy stage, being a part-time caregiver, part-time parent. She sometimes asks about the family, but she can't remember the names of all her kids.

Maybe she sticks her tongue out at me when I leave. I've never dared to look back.

Mom: I miss being around ordinary people.

Me: Mom, you have never liked being around ordinary people.

Mom looks at me and laughs.

Interpreter

Late 2003

Mom's latest complaint: "People are talking about me. I am an adult and I can speak for myself."

She doesn't hear what people say to her, especially in casual conversation. When we go out to eat, a nod will cue her to place an order, but let the server ask if she wants coffee and she is oblivious.

"And how are you ladies tonight?" will often bring the response, "Have you met my daughter?" I've learned not to take it personally. She's not trying to fix me up.

At the doctor's office, it is a different story. On the way to the appointment, she wants to know why she is going and then complains, "I've never set eyes on that man before." Her doctor is a woman, but that doesn't register. She has been here before, but it is all new to her again. I tell her to have a seat in the waiting area while I check her in. It is too much information in one breath.

"Go." I say. "Sit down." Still too much. I point to the chairs.

She says to the receptionist, "I'm here to see the doctor." The receptionist is sitting behind a glass panel. Mom can see her mouth move but cannot hear the words. A little more loudly she says, "I'm here to see the doctor." When she cannot hear the response this time, she turns away from the window and jerks away from me. She goes to the chairs and snatches up a magazine.

Why not let her check herself in? We tried. The glass enclosure is one barrier, but the receptionist is also wearing a headset and answering the phone. Mom can't tell when she is being spoken to. "Tell her to speak up! She's mumbling." Finally Mom is so disgusted she says, "You deal with it. Maybe you can understand what she's flapping her gums about."

The nurse stands at the doorway of the waiting room and calls my mother's name. I look around at the assembled patients. This practice specializes in geriatrics. Most of the patients are at least seventy and older. I bet most are wearing some kind of hearing aid. Why doesn't the nurse come into the room and address patients where they can see and hear her? I notice the younger adults who provide transportation; we are the ones who respond to the nurse. I tap Mom's arm. "They're ready for you."

"What?" She is irritated.

I point to the nurse. "She called your name." Mom gets to her feet. She doesn't want me in the room.

Less than five minutes later, the doctor stands at the door. My mother is behind her with The Look on her face.

I can only imagine the business owners who were on the receiving end of The Look in years past. When she was enforcing civil rights laws, those owners would pay thousands of dollars to make her go away and take her Look with her. I know The Look from childhood, but God help the unsuspecting person who runs into it for the first time.

The doctor asks if I'll come to the exam room and explains that my mother is having difficulty understanding what she is saying.

My mother, who doesn't hear any of this at all, snaps, "Maybe you can make some sense of this. She opens her mouth and nothing comes out." The three of us go back to the exam room and there begins the fine exchange that will collect information without insulting Mom's intelligence.

The doctor sits within arms' reach of Mom, looking her in the eyes, and asks me the question Mom needs to answer. I sit so Mom can see my face and then use my schoolteacher voice to ask the questions. Mom alternates her answers with complaints about the doctor's soft voice and her tendency to mumble. I ignore those parts. The doctor explains some of Mom's concerns to me, but never turns her face away from my mother. I translate. Mom looks surprised. She has *never* had such a problem. She *never* said any such thing.

The doctor is patient. I am exhausted. Mom needs a blood test and seems to understand that. When we stop in the hallway at the lab though, she is confused. "I thought we were done. Let's go. What are we doing here?" She points to the young lab tech and says, "That girl is here every time we come in."

Life is an eight-track tape, and more than one track is audible at any given time. I have my own running commentary that accompanies it all. I want to make this all easier, more efficient. I want to fix it all.

Pay attention to who is around, who is listening, who will need the explanation that I am not a loud-mouthed angry bitch full-time. I am tired of explaining, tired of doing both the advance work and the cleanup.

People have tried a number of tactics so Mom can understand them. When she first moved in, aides wrote notes on a dry erase board. She rejected that outright. "I'm not a child. Talk to me!"

They have written reminder notes. "Your daughter will be here at 4 to go out to dinner." When I show up, she has no idea I was coming. No one told her.

They try talking louder. It doesn't work. Change the batteries in the hearing aids? No, she does it herself every week and won't let anyone else touch them.

What improves her hearing? If she likes the person and is enjoying the conversation. If there's chocolate. If there's a man involved.

In mid-December, I find her helping the Activity Director pack combs and toothbrushes into cellophane bags. They are doing it for residents of a local homeless shelter. "I've been doing this for years," my mother says. Around us, the common area is decorated for the season and I point out a big sign reminding residents of the Family Holiday Dinner the next night. "Tomorrow, okay?" She nods.

Save the Bones

When my sister and I arrive for the dinner the next night, Mom is surprised to see us. She didn't know there was going to be a party or that we were coming. She'd written it on her calendar in three different places. I know she did.

It really isn't about hearing anymore.

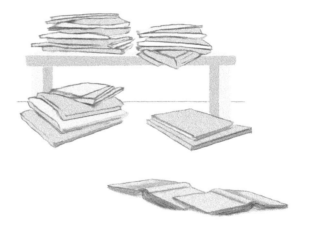

This Ship Never Docks

It is summer 2003. Mom is settled in at an Alzheimer's care facility in Olympia. We have spent so much time getting her settled in, shopping for things, getting her room to be her own. Finally there is time to look around and see the other people who live here. My first impression: there are mostly women here. Not surprising, since women tend to live longer than men. The women are almost uniformly short, their hair neatly permed, and some take great care with lipstick and eyeliner. A few are very well-dressed, as if they plan to go out for the afternoon, perhaps to play cards or enjoy tea. By contrast, my mother is tall, 5'9", has never fussed with her appearance, drinks coffee, and cards bore her.

The few men are shorter than Mom and decently groomed. One wears a bicycle helmet but I have yet to see him on a bike. Another pushes a walker with a calendar hung from the basket. The calendar is permanently set on November 1999. I wonder if that is a particularly important month for him, but he never talks to me or anyone else that I can tell.

The women remind me of girls I knew in high school. They seem to have been friends for decades, though I will find out later that they came from different towns and never went to the same schools. They sit in chatty groups and tell stories about their grandchildren and about their husbands who are all dead, if the stories are to be believed. "The Girls" comment on who is wearing the same outfit the fourth day in a row, who hasn't bothered to set her wig on straight, and make some wild speculation about whether Jack, the latest addition to the population, could handle one or more of them on his—shhhhh—double bed. They keep tabs on who has visitors and who goes out to eat. They talk about their ungrateful children and the bum of a husband their daughter married.

Having left behind their other circles of friends, they gather around each other and slip into familiar conversation. One observes, "Dorothy's not looking so spry today."

"What's that? She was a spy?"

"Not looking SPRY." The puzzled look brings back the spelling trick. "I said, 'She's not s-p-r-y today.'" That doesn't always work but the conversation goes on. "Don't you think so, Kathleen?"

Kathleen, who hasn't been paying attention, jerks her head in the direction of the voice. "What's that? Good day. Is it time for breakfast yet?"

From an annoyed Jackie: "We've had breakfast. And lunch. If you don't watch out, you'll miss dinner altogether, Kathleen."

Kathleen nods. "Yes, I do like this music, Jackie. Reminds me of the first time I met Tony. He's the one I didn't marry." She hums a bit, but because there is no music playing, she loses her place and turns away again.

Jackie rolls her eyes. "Impossible to talk to that one." I wonder how my mother is going to get along with this crowd. Maybe if the batteries in her hearing aids are always fresh, and if she turns the contraptions on, maybe she'll be okay in the conversations.

As I chat with one of the workers, she points out a woman in a pink jogging suit. "She's been here for a couple of years now. Nice lady. You'll see her making the rounds from the common room to the TV room to the garden, almost like clock-work." I watch the almost elegant grace with which the woman greets residents and workers alike. The worker smiles a bit. "She thinks she's on a cruise around the world."

"Doesn't anyone try to tell her where she really is?" I want to know.

"At first, we tried telling her she was in a special facility, to help her memory, but it only made her cry and get agitated. Finally, we decided that she was happy sailing around the world and, as long as she doesn't try to go overboard, we'd let her go on believing that. The ship never docks and we provide everything she needs: meals, a hair salon, a beautiful view." She points to the garden outside in the center of the facility.

I think it sounds complicated. "What happens if you have people with competing fantasies? One on a cruise ship, another herding wild mustangs in Montana?"

The aide laughs. "Hasn't happened yet, though I suppose there'll be a first time one of these days. It could happen."

I shake my head. So many of my conversations with Mom are about getting her into the right time frame. It is Sunday, not Tuesday. It is morning, not evening. Relatives are coming tomorrow, not next week. It is exhausting. But I can't imagine my mother getting stuck thinking she is on a cruise ship.

Alzheimer's has a way of setting a new agenda, of refocusing what is important. I will have to learn to let go of being right. Later, I'll resign myself to sailing on the ship that never docks.

Testing, Testing

There are doors and then there are doors. The door to Mom's room can be locked from the inside or with her key. The door to the hallway that leads to the dining room is always open. And the route to the TV room and the garden is easy to access. (If you keep making a right turn, eventually you end up with food or people.) The door to the front parking lot is a different thing altogether. You must know the code.

In other places, the code will be the numbers of the month and the year, whispered by a nurse or a passing aide—if they're sure you're a member of the public and not a resident trying to escape. Here it's a little more complicated.

A cheerful sign hangs above the keypad. The current code is written in Roman numerals and there is a reminder to punch in the numbers backward. Looking at it, you have to translate the Roman numerals into Arabic ones, and then remember them long enough to punch them into the keypad in reverse.

That's at least two or three steps more than Alzheimer's patients can manage at any one time. Just pushing on the door causes an annoying buzz that must be cancelled by someone at the desk. Visitors become expert at putting in the code and sliding out the door without a resident on their heels.

Mom never notices the sign.

With My Mother

With my mother I have been many people:
    a daughter, certainly,
    the oldest of the bunch,
    the responsible one.

I was a confidant
in the bitter black years
when her (second) marriage was coming apart.
She asked so many questions
and my twelve-year-old self tried to answer.
She never liked my answers,
never followed my advice.

It didn't occur to me to say,
"Why do you think I'd know the answer to this?
Who is the grownup here?"

For a time, I was her first husband,
a man I knew only in a photograph
taken when he'd joined the army.
He was funny, she told me,
exciting,
had a wonderful laugh.
My eyes were like his.
I would stare into his eyes
under the Army cap and try to see my own.
Our noses were more alike.

Then I became the one far away,
away at school, away in Italy, away from home.
By the time I was ready to return,
she had run away,

moved to San Francisco,
and started a new life.

I was the daughter with a job,
with no crazy boyfriends,
no bad habits worth mentioning.
My siblings took up her worry quotient.

We wrote.
We called.
We discussed the family.
"They never write.
They never call," she complained.
Thirty years later, we are still having the same conversation.

In these past years,
I became her interpreter,
taking her to the doctor,
using my schoolteacher voice
to help her understand
what the doctor wants.

I am the front line,
trying to shield her from some big mistake
that would only embarrass me.
(Why does that matter?)

I am the cab driver,
the errand runner,
the Sunday dinner companion,
the family connection.

But last Monday,
I became a smuggler.
Into her room at the nursing home,

where the TV is always on,
tuned to a game show
or an infomercial,
and where she complains
that it is too quiet,
and wonders what we are waiting for,
into her room
I smuggled an ice cream cone:
vanilla ice cream
dipped in chocolate
and rolled in nuts
with a chunk of chocolate
at the point of the cone.

She raised an eyebrow
and bit into it.

Chocolate flaked and nuts flew.
"Oh, that's good," she said.
She ate it all
down to the bottom of the cone.
"I might break my teeth!"
so I took it from her
and peeled away the wafer cone.

"Here, pure chocolate."
She closed her eyes.
Her mouth was ringed with chocolate.
"I'd like some of this for Christmas."

I can do that. A little more smuggling. I can do that.

July 2005

We're Both Changing

We have been to the doctor's, an ordeal of hearing and not hearing. Mom has an infection. It can be cured with a single pill. We go to lunch afterwards. Now, just a mile from her home, I see the drug store and say, "Let's get your prescription filled now." She says, "Good idea." We pull into the parking lot.

The modern drug store isn't very simple. It's a long walk from the front door to the pharmacy. Seasonal sales (post back-to-school and not-quite Halloween) and non-perishable foods have to be navigated. Then the color section: for the hair, the lips, the fingernails. Finally, aspirin and toothpaste and footcare. We are getting closer.

We present the prescription to the pharmacist. It is just a single pill we need. This is going to be easy.

The questions begin.

No, Mom hasn't had any prescriptions filled here before.

"Fill out this information sheet." I take the pen and start writing, but Mom wants to fill it out for herself. I give her the pen.

She stares at the list of questions. "Why do they want to know this?" No explanation helps. "This is an invasion of privacy."

She throws down the pen when she can't remember her new address.

"List your current medications" and I know we are done.

"Never mind," I say to the pharmacist as I take back the prescription, "we'll do this another day. Let's go." I turn away from the counter and look for the exit. I didn't leave bread crumbs when we came in and I'm not too sure I can find my way out again.

"Come back here," my mother yells. I keep going. "Get back here, you bitch. Don't you walk away from me." I turn back. Between clenched teeth I tell her we are going home, that we'll take care of this later. She grabs the paper from my hand and heads back to the pharmacy, sweeping past a display of tuna and crackers that threatens to collapse.

"No." I yank the paper and turn her to the front door. "Later." She follows me, calling me names all the way to the parking lot.

"You are such a bitch. You always have been," she seethes.

I open her door. "Get in." I am furious. I hate scenes in public places. She stands there, refusing to move. "Get in." I go around to the driver's side and get in. I put the keys in the ignition. She gets in the car. Her door hangs open. "Close your door."

"Why?"

"So we can go."

"I don't want to go. I want my pills."

"Later. Close the door." She sits there.

I get out of the car, go around to her side and slam the door. I get back in the car. She grabs the keys from the ignition. I grab them back.

Then she slaps me. I feel a lifetime of slaps.

I jam the keys into the ignition and start the car. I am too angry to drive but too afraid of what I might do if we stay here.

Back at her place, I throw the car into park, jerk the brake, and let her fend for herself getting out. She follows me inside, hissing at my back, still trying to take the prescription from me. By now it is beyond a battle of wills. I am my mother's daughter.

Her anger has always been ferocious. My sister remembers her turning on a dime and exploding over things when we were growing up. I remember matching her volume but never daring to use her swear words. We got into huge arguments when I was a teenager.

The episode in the parking lot undoes me. Inside, I find the nurse and turn over the prescription. My mother complains long and loud that she is capable of caring for herself. I tell all this to long-time aide Peggy. I cry and cry. She listens to me rant, gives me a tissue for the tears, and tells me there will be episodes like this, that Mom is going to keep on changing and I'd better commit myself to not being able to control much of anything anymore. "What has happened to my mother?" I wail.

Mom has no hesitation about being vicious. Sometimes she's very funny, sometimes cruel. It had been a long time since her anger was turned against me and more than thirty years since she slapped me.

Her emotions are raw, on the surface, a throwback to other days. Probably we have done too much for one day. If we'd only seen the doctor and gone to lunch, maybe she could have handled it. Stopping at the drug store was just too much. The breaking points are all too visible with hindsight: having to fill out a form she didn't understand, not getting her questions answered, setting out to do one thing and not finishing it.

I treated her like a child. I didn't give her the form to fill out right away. I'd just taken it and started writing, as if she were incapable. It is one more bit of evidence that she's lost control of something in her life, and I am rubbing her nose in it, making a point of showing her just how much she can't do by herself anymore.

My own lifelong habits have kicked in too. I have to be right, have to show her who is in control. It is ugly. Nothing like having your worst traits on display in a parking lot. Her disease is changing both of us.

Mom is sitting in the lobby when I finally leave. She waves at me and calls, "Goodbye! It was good to see you today!"

Thanksgiving

Thanksgiving dinner. Turkey and all the trimmings: mashed potatoes, gravy, cranberry sauce, vegetables. Family tradition, of sorts. Mom hasn't cooked Thanksgiving dinner since the early '70s. My sister and I vote for expediency. Neither of us wants to cook and Mom maxes out at two hours. We'll let someone else cook and do the dishes.

Easy enough. The newspaper is full of ads, plenty of restaurants offering Thanksgiving meals. It's just a matter of finding one.

Not just finding one. Finding one that can cater to Mom being a vegetarian. She doesn't eat turkey.

We settle on Falls Terrace in Olympia with its dining room that overlooks the local waterfall. It is a destination restaurant, the place where anniversaries are celebrated and engagements settled, home of great reunions.

We join the line at the appointed time and are seated quickly. Special menus are handed around. Mom scans the list: turkey, prime rib, salmon. She slaps the menu down. "Well, there's nothing here for me to eat!"

The man overseeing the staff comes to the table immediately and asks how he might help. We explain, or try to. Mom goes on and on about the backwardness of businesses that refuse to acknowledge the rising tide of vegetarians.

The man bows. He promises her something wonderful from the kitchen.

It is noisy in the restaurant, but no place would have been quiet enough for a good conversation. We let Mom take the lead; if she asks questions or makes a comment, she is feeling up to responding without too much repetition.

Erin and I have mastered the technique of carrying on our own conversation while looking in another direction.

Before Mom can start complaining again about the plethora of meat-eaters, dinner comes to the table. Our server presents an exquisite plate of vegetables, built on mashed potatoes, with cranberry sauce on the side.

"Where did this come from?" Mom demands as she pokes her fork into the creation.

"They made it especially for you," Erin explains.

"Why?"

"Because they know you are a vegetarian and they wanted you to have a special meal today."

Mom frowns but takes a bite of the steaming vegetables.

Eventually she makes a point of asking the server to thank the cooks for such a good meal. She thanks the manager for his help.

After pie and coffee, we get up from the table, another Thanksgiving meal behind us. But Mom gets agitated about the bill. We are paying at the cash register, but she doesn't understand. She stands next to the table, arguing. Nothing we say can convince her that we are not walking out without paying.

I leave Erin to deal with her and go to pay the bill. The lobby is crowded, more families wanting to celebrate the big day. A few peer into the dining room and look at the woman who is refusing to leave. I want to yell, "It's Alzheimer's, okay? I wish I could fix it and make her normal but get this: she has never been normal! Be glad she's not your mother." But I don't. I pay the bill. She comes to the register and wants to argue. I tell her the bill is paid. It is time to go. We make our way through the crowd between the cash register and the door.

"You're a bitch," she says to my back.

Erin tries to calm her. "Mom." Her reasoned voice has no effect. Mom goes into a full-blown name-calling tirade. "Where did you learn to act like this?" she yells.

"I got it from you!"

We take her back home. She shakes off our goodbyes. "I hope they're serving something good tonight. I haven't eaten anything for hours."

"Too bad we don't drink," my sister says as we drive out of the parking lot.

"Yeah, too bad."

A cheer Mom taught us kids:

Shelby, Shelby, we think you're IT!

S-H for Shelby, I-T for IT!

The New Place

Winter 2004

It begins, as it often does, with a phone call from a nurse. "Your mother has been talking about moving. She doesn't want to do any activities because she is moving. She wonders what it will be like at the new place she is moving to." Is she moving? No.

She's not moving. I thought we had settled this. But there is no "we" with Alzheimer's.

Over dinner, Mom explains that the staff told her that she doesn't need to stay here. "The medicines have improved me so much, I can move to a new place!"

I shake my head. "You're not moving." She is adamant. The staff told her she is well enough to move.

I remind her of the talk she had with the staff before Christmas, how they had asked for suggestions, wanted to know what they could improve. She was full of ideas then. They planned on having her stay.

"I'm not moving?"

"No, you're not moving."

"Oh, thank God. I couldn't stand the thought of moving again." She still hasn't hung the pictures we sent home with her at Christmas. Someone offered to hang them, but she told him not to bother because she was moving.

She acknowledges that she forgets things. "Is my memory problem very noticeable?"

"Only when we talk about moving," I say.

"Have we talked about that tonight?"

"A number of times."

She hoots and laughs and throws her arms into the air. "I'm moving, right?"

"No, you're not moving. You have moved for the last time."

"Thank God."

Later that evening she calls. "I just wanted to ask you what the new place is like."

"There is no new place, Mom. You are not moving."

"I'm not?"

"No. You can stay there till you decide to drop."

She chews on this for a while. "They aren't kicking me out?"

"No, they like you. If you start beating on other residents, they might ask you to think about a new place."

I can hear her thinking. She asks, "What about a few well-placed kicks?" I laugh. "I need some new shoes," she announces, "with steel toes. When we go shopping next time, that's what I want."

"Okay, Mom."

She promises to hang the pictures the next day. She is not moving.

The Day Aunt Alley Came to Stay

Once upon a time... *(Sometimes fiction is the only way to grapple with new situations.)*

Nobody warned us. Although our extended family had long histories of relatives who came for a visit and stayed for years, no one warned us.

In our grandparents' generation, their parents lived with them until death. People died at home, especially relatives. They died at home.

One of my grandmothers cared for her in-laws in Seattle while her husband disappeared into New York City back in the thirties.

The other cared for her older brother when he went blind again in his later years.

When I was growing up, Uncle Ed came to stay in our utility room. He had just the bed and a desk with an old typewriter. He wrote stories about Damon Runyon-type characters, including the memorable Horizontal Helen. (One of his sisters, in a fit of family decorum, burned the existing manuscripts. Helen remains in memory only.)

Aunt Alley was a surprise. She showed up like some carpetbagger, her hair three weeks past due for a perm. Her green eye shadow and penciled-on brows made us look twice. Just where were her eyes anyway? She'd applied her rouge without looking, so the colored marks did not exactly match on her cheeks. Her lipstick was applied precisely but the shade was known only to the back bins at Goodwill.

If we'd seen her coming down the street, I'm sure we would have tagged after her, yelling inane things, but, as it was, no one saw her coming.

She knocked on our front door and I opened it. She bit a cigarette holder between her teeth. (We found out later that she'd given up smoking, but not the holder.) "Hey, girlie," she greeted me, "is your mother home?"

"Um, well, I, Mom!" I babbled. The woman shoved her duffle bag through the door and it thunked on the hardwood floor. Three big clunky bracelets rattled around her wrist. They didn't match. She stopped to look at me and sniffed, "I've heard about you, girlie." She thumped my head with her bracelets and came into the living room. Her straw purse overflowed and a hole in the bottom corner threatened to expel everything.

My mother came from the kitchen, wiping her hands on a dish towel. "What's all the noise?" She looked at the visitor and then looked at me.

"She asked for you," I said, shrugging my shoulders.

The woman grabbed my mother's hand and shook it. "Alyce, my dear. I'm your Aunt Alyce." She took the cigarette holder out of her mouth and stuck it behind her ear. "Twice removed, on your mother's side. Can you be removed twice? No matter. I'm here now. You can call me Alley."

By this time a crowd had grown in the living room. My sister appeared from her bedroom. Three of the brothers arrived with their neighborhood buddies in tow, bikes at rest in the driveway. The youngest brother was still trapped in his high chair but was capable of going great distances.

"Aunt, umm, Alley," my mother said faintly, "won't you come in?" She gestured to the couch and Aunt Alyce plopped down.

We kids stared. Her tennis shoes were bright orange with green laces. She wore socks festooned with red hearts. Her pants might have been paisley once but were so faded it was hard to tell for sure. The blouse was finely tailored with well-pressed pleats and she wore two pins on the collar, "LBJ in '64" and "Viva la huelga!"

Mom took a deep breath. "So you're from my mother's side of the family?"

"Yep," said Alley, "not that I've talked to any of them recently."

"It's just that, well, I don't remember anyone ever mentioning you." My normally poised mother was finding it hard to speak.

Aunt Alyce barked. "Ha! Not likely that they'd mention Crazy Alley, is it?" She laughed at her own joke then dug into her purse and pulled out a cigarette case. "Smokes, anyone?" She flipped open the case. The boys pushed forward.

"No!" my mother protested, but Aunt Alyce passed the case around. Soon every kid under ten was smoking a candy cigarette.

"Okay, calm down," Aunt Alyce said to Mom. "Won't hurt them." Mom opened her mouth and then closed it. She shut her eyes and sat down.

And so crazy Aunt Alley moved in, shoving aside basic family mess and noise, making herself one with the local chaos. She did not resemble Grandma or her side of the family. They were all sturdy solemn characters who lined up for pictures at family picnics in the late forties. The women wore skirts or dresses with long sleeves. Everyone wore a hat. There were no children in the pictures—or at least no child-aged children. The lineup was always the great-grandparents and their adult children. Looking at the photos again, I wondered who had taken the pictures. Was that how they kept Crazy Alley out of sight? Put her behind the camera instead of into the line?

Telling Time

January/February 2005

Since she moved to Washington from California, keys have become Mom's measuring stick. This week, she wears her room key on a gold chain around her neck. Last week, she told me, "They won't give me a key, no matter how often I ask. They don't trust me," she complained.

She has had several keys. At first she wore a key on a metal ring threaded through her watch band. She'd worn a key that way for years, even when she was in Santa Barbara. It was always at hand, no fear of losing it.

When she moved to this place in Olympia, her new key went on the watchband again. She was meticulous about locking her door. Unlike her old apartment at the end of a hallway on the third floor, now her room is steps away from the TV room where people come and go all day. She is wary of wanderers who might have sticky fingers.

In the past few months, things have changed. The key comes and goes. Sometimes she slips the metal ring around her finger. One day she had a new key on a plastic coil with her name written on a small plastic heart. She wore it like a bracelet around her wrist, and later, shoved it to the upper part of her arm. The other key, the one she'd lost, lay in a case on her night stand, next to the hearing aid batteries I am sure she no longer remembers to change.

One night, when we'd had dinner in the small side dining room, I got ready to leave. "But what about me?" she asked. "Aren't you going to take me home?"

"You are home, Mom. You live here."

"I do?" She was incredulous. "Since when?" She sat down with a thump. "I have never lived here."

"You've been here almost two years," I explained.

"But I don't know anyone! I couldn't tell you the name of a single person here." I thought to remind her of Simon. She introduces me to him every time I come.

This is one of the deep sorrows she knows now. A woman with many friends in her lifetime and with a gift for talking to anyone, now she lives with people who pull inward, who do not respond to her. Deafness plays a role. She cannot hear the voices of the soft-spoken women. She says they all stayed home, never went to work, let their husbands do all the talking, and now they are boring and have nothing to say. Arguing with her is beside the point.

She doesn't hear from many old friends. She was once a champion letter writer and phone caller. One old co-worker from San Francisco writes to her now from Switzerland. Sometimes she writes back, but she doesn't remember. She hasn't used long distance in months, not even to call me. It is a relief of sorts. She had been calling me in the middle of the night to check the time.

Alzheimer's has pulled her into herself in ways she cannot see.

It's not about the keys, but it is. No key can turn back the time; no key will unlock the door to the future she once hoped for. This is not what she imagined. Her parents traveled well into their eighties, and after her mother died, her father still made the trip from Tacoma to Santa Barbara. She imagined old age as a time to travel and explore. Her world has become very small. She has one key. It opens her room but will not let her out the front door.

She does not seem to notice from one moment to the next, but then she gets a look on her face, the look that says she does know. The fear and anger overwhelm her. She knows for a moment what is still yet to come. And she disappears into a place where I cannot reach her.

Worker: Marie, you have a visitor!

Marie: Whiskers? When did that happen?

The Raging of the Shrew

January 2004

Alzheimer's has made me a shrew. I've always been mouthy, but kept it to the people just around me in the classroom or at a meeting. Alzheimer's has made me go public.

Maybe I shouldn't give all the blame to Alzheimer's. I am in the store with Mom, poking at some this or that. She turns down an aisle—or I do—and I lose sight of her. Next time I find her, she is standing, always looking in the opposite direction.

"Mom." No response.

"Mom!" a little louder. Nothing. A woman goes by, pushing her cart. She looks at me when I raise my voice another notch. "Mom!" I look at the woman. "It's like having kids," I say. She looks bewildered. Mom is getting agitated. I can tell by the way she stands, how she shifts on her feet. She is not hearing me (has she replaced her hearing aid batteries recently?). She is ignoring me. My voice isn't registering as someone she knows. Maybe I should call her by her first name. The woman and her cart move on.

I go to my mother and put my hand on her shoulder. I turn her to face me. "Mom? Did you find what you need?"

She holds up a pair of funny socks and says, "I was looking for some hand cream."

Alzheimer's has changed our relationship. Mom and I had gotten to a point, back in the early eighties, where I'd finally convinced her that I couldn't be my dead father, her first husband, Bob. He was the great love of her life, and since this last move, the one great memory she has. He died when they were both young. He was 25 and she was two months shy of 24. They married in 1951, went through a miscarriage, had me in 1953, and two weeks later found out he had cancer. He was dead the next June.

With the wisdom of the time, she remarried fifteen months later and eventually had five more children. That marriage came apart in the early seventies. From the time I was twelve, she told me I was all she had left of the best love of her life.

In the 1980s, she was working for the state of California in civil rights enforcement. It was fun to visit her, to hear about her cases, to cheer the big victories like the first AIDS discrimination case. She lived in San Francisco and then Anaheim. Her last assignment was in Ventura where she owned a couple of properties and lived in a four-plex where the upstairs was always being remodeled.

She loved second-hand stores and found fabulous doorknobs, tiles, lamp stands, chairs. As often as I'd visit, it was always a work in progress. She lived without a stove or an oven, making dinner on a two-burner hot plate with rare excursions into the microwave.

After she retired, she moved to an apartment in Santa Barbara. She was all over the city at political rallies, art exhibitions, movies, the symphony. Her letters were full of clippings from the newspapers.

She retired because her hearing had deteriorated and working on the phone became too difficult.

But it was also after her retirement that we began to notice changes. Always a confident driver, now there were near misses. She left coffee to burn on the stove. Was it just forgetfulness? She didn't care what day it was. She was retired and didn't need to know. They seemed to be such minor things.

There were arguments with long-time friends that she didn't patch up. We'd ask about someone she'd known for years and there would be a flood of complaints or a dismissive, "We don't have much in common."

Talking to her took energy. She couldn't hear (when had I learned to mumble?), she didn't remember the plans we'd made. I'd spent my childhood listening to adults yelling and now having to yell to make myself heard, I felt mad at her all the time—and only because I had to raise my voice.

Every call, every visit, became an inquiry, a chance for diagnosis. Was she really different? Was I seeing something new? My brother, who saw her more often, reassured me that there wasn't anything unusual going on. I just kept adding to my mental list.

Eventually, with Geoff's help, she moved to a retirement home, a renovated dorm that once belonged to the University of California at Santa Barbara. After my initial visit, my sister and I decided that we would not do another visit alone. It took both of us to share the energy needed to keep her on track or to distract her when she was "caught in the loop."

A final visit and we knew that we were the upset in her routine, that some of her behavior happened because we were there. At the same time, people began to report other problems they were seeing. It became clear another move needed to happen.

And that's about the time the eviction notice came.

She called several times to say she was being evicted. Other residents were being evicted too, she said. They were going to file a lawsuit claiming discrimination, but they couldn't figure out the common factor. She was an expert in these things. What had she spent the last years working on? Civil rights enforcement! She called me. She called my brother. I called my brother. What's going on?

With some effort, we pieced it together. Geoff had written her a letter outlining why she should think about moving. He and his wife had moved away from Santa Barbara and there was no longer family close by. If she moved to Washington, she'd at least have her two daughters and some grandchildren. She needed a different place. She read that as her eviction letter. We began to make plans.

Years past that point, I can understand now that we were witnessing the fraying of fabric, the gentle coming apart at the worn places. Incidents and people were too new to stay with her. They slid like soap bubbles and were gone.

How to deal with it? Sometimes the questions get repeated within a short span. It is exhausting. I begin to feel like the village idiot. Am I not being clear? When Erin and I visit her together, we're a tag team, each giving the other respite, distracting her with something different. Alone with her, I try to stay in the moment until she is caught in the loop again. Then it is time to break the connection. Yesterday that meant visiting for only twenty minutes.

She manages two good hours out of her comfort zone. If I take her out, we do only two things, no more. She is overloaded and gets mean when she has gone too long. At Christmas, two hours were enough to have a good meal and appreciate presents. Though she seemed to be doing well, we knew the forty-minute trip back to her place would put her on edge. My brother drove her home and she dismissed him, even though he'd brought new pictures to hang on her wall. She was done. He could go.

Me: Hi, Mom. It's my birthday. I brought you some ice cream.

Mom: Congratulations! When and where were you born?

Me: In Seattle, 1953.

Mom: I was born in Seattle.

Me: I know. And you grew up in Tacoma.

Mom: How did you know that?

Me: Because you're my mother. And you told me.

Mom eats the ice cream. The look on her face says, "I'll be polite but I don't have a clue what you're talking about."

On Notice

I find my pockets full of scraps of conversations with my mother. Is she feeding me lines for a stand-up routine? Sometimes I think so.

She says, "I'm going to sue them." And when I ask why, she says, "Improper supervision of the inmates!" The nursing home won't be pleased, I think, but she may be on to something.

She makes her rounds and stops at the front desk. The receptionist looks at her and smiles. "Good morning, Marie. What's new?"

Mom edges closer to the desk, leans over it, and lowers her voice. "I'll tell you what's new." She looks over her shoulder and confides, "That man came in my room again. He wanted to borrow a book. When I said no, he peed in my wastebasket."

The woman at the desk looks shocked.

Mom grunts in satisfaction. "Can't be tolerated," she says, "can't be tolerated. I'm going to sue."

"You should," says the woman at the desk, "that's just wrong."

On Valentine's Day, Mom asks, "Did we eat with the prince?" Later, "I haven't had a good romantic relationship in a long time," a Jack Benny pause, "or a bad one." I swallow my laughter, but only for a moment. We both laugh.

Out in the TV room, wrapped in a blanket, Mom waves her arm beckoning for service. "Where is my ticket?" she wants to know. "What time does my plane leave?" There aren't any answers.

I'm betting she'll be suing the airlines next.

Voices from the Past

The voice on the tape is tired, almost a whisper. "It's been a long tough road," the man says, "but we managed to cram a lifetime into three years." I close my eyes and try to see him, lying on a bed in the afternoon, blankets pulled up around him. He has the microphone of a reel to reel tape recorder in his hand. He's talking to my mother. He tells her he loves her. My uncle tells me that his brother had lost a lot of weight fighting the cancer. He is rail thin in the 1953 Christmas pictures.

The tape recorder provided some entertainment for them. There's a party sequence, with "bouquets prepared by the Washington State Liquor Board," according to my mother who announces the event. "Little Brown Jug" plays in the background. These people like to laugh.

There is a brief bit that sounds like it came from the McCarthy hearings: "I have proof that you are a communist. You're on the list of subscribers for the *People's Daily World*." Later, there is a long discussion about Senator Joseph McCarthy's tactics and a brisk debate about people being called "Fifth Amendment Communists."

A few seconds of the tape are directed to me. "You were just in here a while ago. Stop screaming." A sharp scream comes from the kitchen. "You're cute anyway. I don't know where you got that scream. Maybe your mom should move you to Iowa and you could win a few hog-calling contests." The affection in his voice is unmistakable. The voice is a counterpoint to the only picture I had of him when I was growing up. His Army picture looked so formal.

"Love you. Lots much."

For Sale

It's a funky house in an otherwise conservative neighborhood. With two stories built of wood like some of the others down the street, its foundation is like many constructed at the same time. They mix well with the brick houses that exude permanence and well-being.

The house sits well on its lot; a straightforward walkway leads from the sidewalk to the three steps going up to the porch. There is a swing on the porch, wide enough for one to lie down with a good book and a glass of lemonade, one leg dangling to the floor for the occasional push. Departures do not happen quickly here.

The hedge by the sidewalk has always been about waist high to kids. There's a permanent dip in it where the challenge to jump cannot be resisted. The sharp clear lines have blurred with age, but the hedge still frames the yard near the sidewalk.

Down the street, gardens are tidy and predictable. Crocus, daffodil, tulip, iris appear in seasonal waves. At this house, a cacophony of color erupts with no warning, splashing blue and purple amid orange and six kinds of green. Red visits each season but always in a different part of the garden. Sometimes it is strawberries. Every other year it is apples.

The grass is shaggy, worn in spots, well-trampled over time. Some patches surrendered long ago and refuse to present themselves again. Others are oblivious to time and season.

The house wears a coat of paint four shades brighter than the neighborhood palette, a yellow that brings to mind an old Beatles song or the bird from Sesame Street. The windows are trimmed in a dark currant red, except for the upstairs bedroom window that sports a rainbow around its frame. Seen from across the street, the house winks.

Off and on, a "For Rent" sign appears in the yard, a crisp sign with succinct information. The house settles in on itself, but then the sign comes down.

Lately, there is a new sign. "For Sale." Not an offer of temporary habitation any longer; this is more permanent. The owner is moving.

My mother is that house. She has always been an unexpected find in a conservative neighborhood, out of step with her non-union, Republican parents who did not understand why she wanted to go to college but supported her anyway.

She read authors they never encountered, traveled places they refused to acknowledge (her trip to Japan in the mid-90s would have killed her mother if she hadn't been dead already), and worked at jobs that helped "those people."

She lives now, fiercely independent, scolding or dismissing those who think to limit her. She doesn't understand women of her generation who never worked beyond their own homes. Those women chide her for "talking to men." She is continually amazed by their small world.

The "For Rent" sign began to appear in her life ten years ago. Little cracks showed in the walls of a still-sound house. At first we thought it was just her hearing that was failing. But other things happened. There were moments of disconnect. She forgot a name, a conversation, an opinion. Invited out to dinner, she ate with friends in the dining room of her retirement home. Later, she picked at her food in the restaurant and said, "I'm never hungry anymore."

More recently, the "For Sale" sign hangs in her eyes. She talks of moving, swears she's staying, she has already moved, she will never move. I wait for the day the place is abandoned and closes itself for good. It seems inevitable. We've been to the garage sales here too often. Surely there can't be much left to pack.

Do they put signs on property like "Abandoned by Owner"? Or do they just board up the doors and windows and paint "No Trespassing"?

Originally written 2/14/03, the winter before Mom moved from California to Washington

Marie: I know that woman.

I've seen her before

and it has nothing to do with the belching.

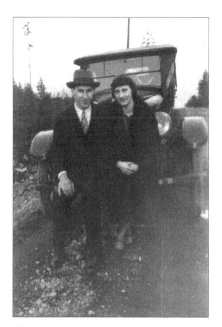

Snazzy hat, snazzy car: Marie's parents Ted and Mary Ultsch in 1926.

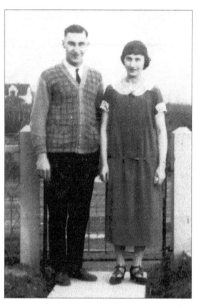

Ted and Mary in 1929 before Marie joined the family.

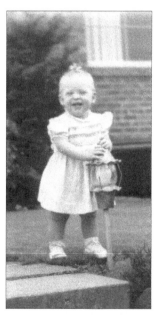

Grandpa took lots of pictures. Lots.

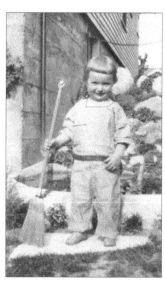

This photo was used in the family's 1932 Christmas card.

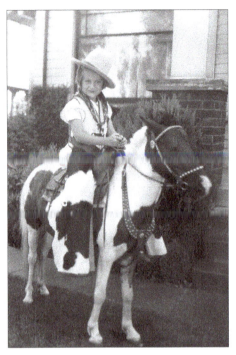

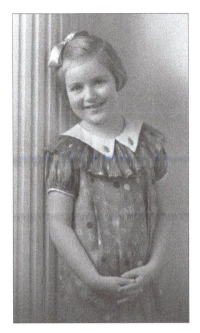

Marie, about age 8 or 9.

1936, photo taken by a photographer who brought his own pony and riding clothes.

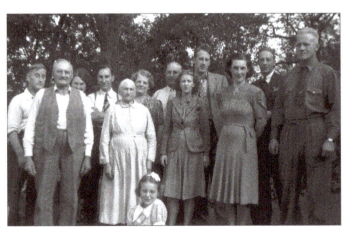

Early 1940s, Sunday picnic in the park with aunts, uncles, and maternal grandparents. Marie is in the front.

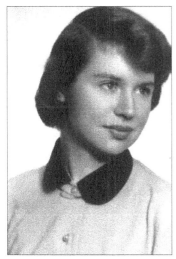
Marie, high school graduation, 1948

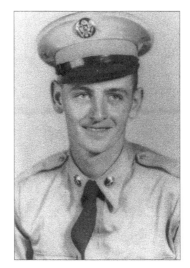
Bob, Army, 1950

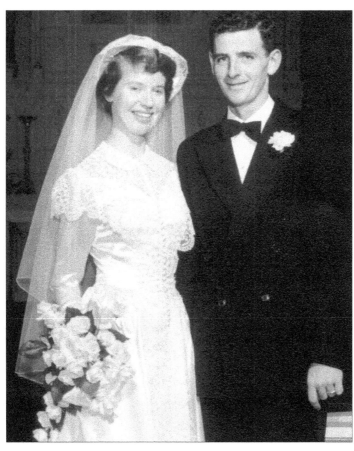
Marie and Bob O'Donnell, September 18, 1951

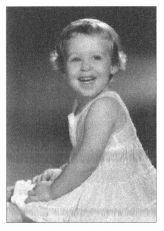

Shannon 1955

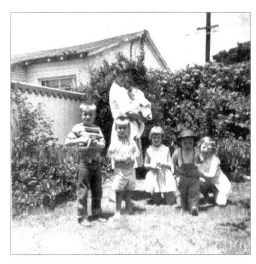

Spring 1963, Marie holding Crispin. In front, James, Theo, Erin, Geoff, Shannon

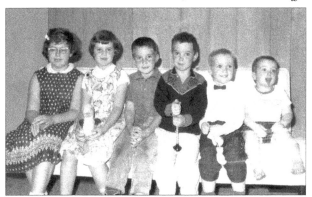

Family line up, Shannon, Erin, James, Theo, Geoff, Crispin . . .

and in reverse order

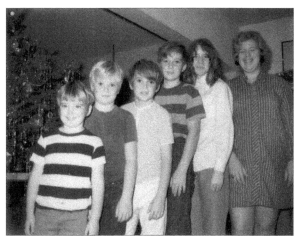

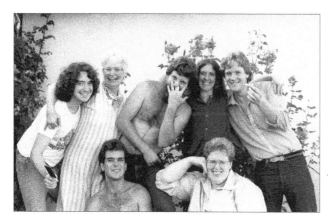

In the mid-80s, we finally moved out of chronological order. From the left, Crispin, Marie, James, Erin, Geoff. Down in front, Theo and Shannon

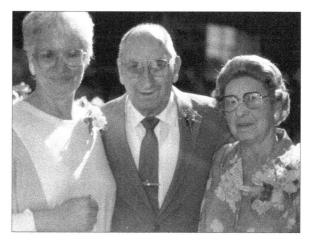

Marie with her parents, Ted and Mary, celebrating their 60 years of marriage.

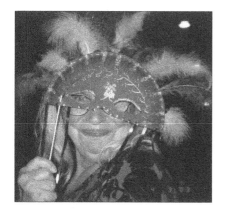

Marie celebrates Mardi Gras

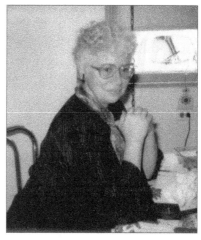

Marie at work, early 1990s

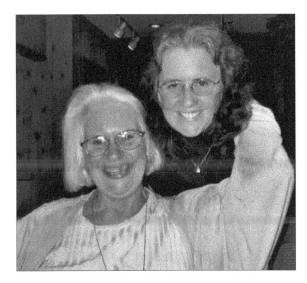

Marie and Erin, Thanksgiving 2003

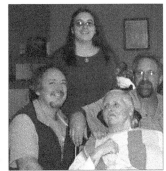

Marie turns 80, with Crispin and his wife Tamar, and James, 2010

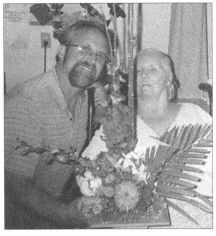

James and Marie, 2012

Part II:
Be Here Now

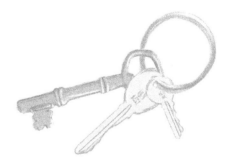

Down Catastrophe Road

Mom is declining. All of a sudden, or so it seems, she has a hard time walking. She grabs my arm if she needs to go from one place to another, even if it is only a few steps. Her hands shake when she uses them. She is unsure. She sleeps most of the day and needs help getting up and dressed. The staff says she can't find her way to her room from the dining room. They have found her staring out the window, not confused, just blank. She wants to know where the kid went. Which kid? "Mine, of course!" For the strong vigorous woman she was, these are huge changes. I don't know what I expected, but this isn't it.

We plan another trip to the doctor. Maybe the meds need readjusting. Much of the change happened since Christmas. There are hallucinations now too. She complains about another resident who kept hearing children crying. Who does Mom see? Does she go back to 1954 with Bob newly dead and me a year old, crying?

We go over old stories. I know some of them, but she surprises me with new versions of others. When I was growing up, I knew she was adopted. It had been a big secret, one kept from her for years. The story I'd heard first was that she was twelve when some neighborhood kid broke the news to her. All the extended family knew, but it explained so many things, including why she didn't resemble any of the relatives.

"My best friend, Joanne, was part of a big Irish family. I loved spending time at her house. It was always busy and noisy. I wanted to be Irish." Mom's family was German-Austrian, already several generations into the American fabric. Mom was devastated to find out she was adopted, she said, but there was a surprise. Her parents showed her the adoption papers, and right there, on the page, was her birth name: Margaret McDonald. Her mother's name was Margaret O'Mara. She was Irish after all.

Now she tells me a different story. She was engaged to my father. The wedding was two months away. Her parents sat her down and broke the news to her. "You're adopted." It took her a week to write to Bob who was away doing training with the Army, a week filled with fear that he wouldn't want to marry her. But he had no problem with it and two young Irish people got married on a September day in 1951.

The big secret of her adoption, however she learned of it, was not to repeat itself in my generation. I had no memories of my father. From the time I was very young, I had a picture of him in my room and I knew about him. He'd died before I was a year old. When Mom remarried, she made a point of explaining to each of my siblings why I had an extra grandmother. I always included my father's name into my own.

These days, we spend a lot of time talking about him. It is almost as if her second marriage didn't happen, though there are certainly children to prove that it did. On her bookshelf is a very bad photocopy of her first wedding picture.

This physical frailty has happened so quickly. Is this the final decline? She has been here less than a year. Why this? Why now?

I switch into preparation mode. Where will the funeral be? How will we get the family here? Who needs to be notified? The list gets long.

You notice the first question? About the funeral? That's how quickly I go to Catastrophe. It doesn't take long and I don't need much encouragement. Of course this is going to be very bad. The rest of the chatter in my head is something along the line of, "I'm the oldest. I'm the responsible one. I should be in charge. I know how this is done." On and on.

Truth is: Mom's meds get adjusted and she gets better. No need to file the obituary. This time. Do I learn from this? Of course not.

Hallucinations

—She's being evicted.
—Someone hit her.
—A man climbed into her bed.

At first I didn't know how to take her stories. The staff told me about the man in her bed. They investigated. There was a man on staff that night, recently returned from vacation, someone Mom hadn't gotten to know much. But he was assigned to the opposite side of the facility and was caring for another resident. Witnesses had seen him and talked with him. There are no male residents in her section. Still, a report was made so there is a record.

"Sometimes my dreams are very real," Mom says.

This spring she saw her mother chatting with new friends. "Not those old biddies from her church days, better ones." She likes the new place where her mother lives. It seems silly (or cruel) to remind her that Grandma has been dead since 1988.

One of the residents carries a life-like baby doll, rocking and cuddling it. Another has a menagerie of stuffed animals. Depending on the day or the mood, she favors the tiger or the giraffe. She will have nothing to do with the man who fawns over his stuffed dog.

Mom's hallucinations seem more self-oriented. Her deafness had become a problem at Santa Barbara. Here, she says, no one has ever said an unkind word to her.

They have. She hasn't heard. As aggravating as her deafness is, it can be a gift.

I Am Not Who I Think I Am

Mom and I are sitting in a Mexican restaurant in Olympia. It's Mother's Day and we are talking about her mother, my grandmother. "She has much better friends now," my mother says. "Not like those old biddies who used to sit around her living room and play cards once a month. Much more interesting."

"Really." I'm impressed. Grandma's been dead since 1988 but clearly she's in a better neighborhood these days. Mom is enthused. This development has given her new respect for her mother.

Later, Mom asks, "Where is Jacqui these days?"

"In California," I say.

"That's too bad." She takes a long sip of her coffee and sets the cup down. She gives me The Look. "You know, you really should try harder to reconcile with her."

I open my mouth to say something and then realize that Mom thinks I am my brother Geoff who is still happily married to Jacqui and living with her in California.

"You really should try," she says again. I nod and promise to try.

The Hospital: Round One

October 2004

"What are we waiting for?" Mom is impatient. Earlier in the afternoon, she'd fallen in the TV room. She arrived at the hospital in an ambulance and I left work early to meet her. The emergency staff had taken her for an x-ray and now we wait. "Let's get out of here," Mom says. She is sitting up on a gurney and looking out into the busyness of the emergency room. She makes a move to get down.

"Mom." I put a hand on her wrist. "Mom, we have to wait. They're coming back to tell us what's wrong." She shakes off my hand, annoyed at the explanation.

"What's wrong?" she asks. "Where are we? I don't like this place. That man is here every time I come in." She makes a face at the kid whose motorcycle had a brief encounter with a tree. The kid doesn't see her.

"We're at the hospital."

"Why?"

"You fell."

A doctor pulls the curtain behind him as he comes in with the x-ray. He introduces himself and says, "Well, we know what's wrong now." Her hip is broken. She'll have surgery at three. She is out of recovery and in her own room by five. She is chatty when I see her again in the evening.

"Where are we?"

"At the hospital."

"Who's sick?"

"You are. You broke your hip. You had an operation."

"I did?"

"You did."

"Who pushed me?"

"No one pushed you. You fell."

Mom frowns and looks out the window. It's a great view here on the ninth floor. Beyond the parking lot are tall evergreens. The sky is dotted with clouds that refuse to give any hint of rain. "Where am I?"

We go through the conversation again. While she sleeps, I write notes on paper towels. "You are in the hospital."

"Your hip is broken."

"You are okay."

"Stay in bed."

My sister arrives the next day. Mom puts on her Pleasant Smile for Strangers, but it is clear she doesn't know who this new person is. Erin brings a new deck of cards with her. We haven't played 500 since Grandpa was in the hospital more than twelve years ago. This is what we do at the hospital: we play 500. It takes us a while to remember the rules, but Erin beats me anyway.

Mom naps and then asks where she is, why she's here, has the surgery already happened. We answer the questions. We point out the answers on the paper towels that blanket her bed, but Mom ignores them. It is exhausting.

The nurses are very patient with her. They admire the Halloween headband she is wearing with pumpkins bobbing on small springs. She smiles and asks if Christmas is coming soon. But her mood changes suddenly. When a nurse on the late shift comes in to check on her, Mom is startled and belligerent and nasty. When I try to apologize, he shakes his head. "Don't worry about it. The first few days after surgery are always weird."

Over another hand of cards, Erin and I talk about other incidents where Mom acted oddly. There was that family reunion with in-laws at the beach on the Central California coast. Mom had a motel room nearby and planned to spend a few days with some of the grandchildren. She went to the picnic but left early. Then she got in her car and drove home without telling anyone.

A few years later, there was a disastrous Christmas, hurt feelings all around. When she told the story, it was never easy and she'd say she was kicked out, no one would give her anything to eat. I doubt we would have been able to do much back then because she was still so independent. But it makes me wonder just when Alzheimer's made its first appearance in her life.

After a week in the hospital, we discover the limits of the hospital staff. Mom's been yelling. She doesn't like the food. The doctor never visits. She hasn't seen her children in months. Her hip is not broken.

More than one nurse has scolded her for making so much noise and upsetting the other patients on the floor. "You have to settle down! You're making other people cry."

"Prove it," Mom dares her. "You people never listen to me. No one answers my questions." She moves to a dementia facility that can provide rehabilitation for her hip. She is not doing well.

She doesn't sleep much at night. She can't remember that she had surgery. She tries to get up and walk. She screams at the staff. She tosses her food tray. She tries to hit people with her walker.

The consulting nurses from Mental Health recommend a short stay at a psychiatric ward where they specialize in geriatrics. I worry this means that she's headed for the state mental hospital, but a nurse reassures me. "In five years, I've only sent one person to the state hospital and he had a long history of mental illness. That's not your mother's problem. The time at the psych ward will give her a chance to recuperate and get her meds adjusted."

Maybe it's just the meds that need adjusting. On the other hand, if Mom's coping skills have been stripped away because of the fall and the surgery, this may be a more accurate picture of how the disease is affecting her now.

In the hallway, a woman in fuzzy green slippers shuffles by, chanting, "Bok choy! Bok choy!"

Four weeks after breaking her hip, Mom goes home to Olympia. She spent a week in the hospital after her surgery, then three weeks at the psych ward. When I pull the car into the driveway and help her out, she says, "Thanks for the ride. It was nice to go out." She doesn't remember a thing about any of it.

Later she breaks down and wails, "I don't want to die!" She rethinks and corrects herself, "I don't want to depress you."

I try to reassure her. "You can talk about it if you want."

"That's part of family, isn't it?"

It is. We go on. Thanksgiving passed us by. Christmas is a month away.

Notes from a Stay in Rehab

Inside the front cover of the 4" by 4" notebook is my mother's name, Marie Cain. At first glance, it might seem like her signature, but it isn't. That's my handwriting. The 'M' has her familiar swoop, and the lower case 'r' is in her script, but I haven't retained her elegant Greek 'e' and that is what gives it away. When I was in high school, I could imitate her signature well, but I didn't. If I was legitimately absent from school, she wrote the note. If I'd cut class, the note had Dad's name on it.

Room 109

Mom's out of the hospital after her hip surgery. She'll be here for a few weeks getting back on her feet. She's having a hard time hearing, so the notebook is a way for the aides to communicate with her.

Punctuation and spelling aren't in much demand, but the handwriting is clear.

Assist Living
You hurt your hip
so we have to take care of you

This is a constant struggle for Mom. She doesn't remember being in the hospital to start with, doesn't connect the pain she feels with an actual break, and can't remember from one hour to the next what she'd been told about what happened to her.

Do you want to sit in here or lay down
Breakfast 8:00 am
Lunch 12:00 noon
7:00 AM

This last is in larger figures, circled, and underlined half a dozen times. Mom was awake and hungry. Her watch was somewhere else and the clock in the room didn't make sense to her.

The nurse is coming
It is coated *(most likely her medications, not the nurse)*
That should help

The cook said
the food will be
done in a few
minutes

Relax for a while
We will get you better

Why are you crying
You live here now
Shannon will be here today after work

This refrain seems to help. I imagine the aides chanting it as they work with her or maybe piling curses on my head. It is always evening when I come. She's had a long day, her energy is gone, things are more confusing.

Your roomate name is Alice
She's very nice.

Did I mention Mom hates having a roommate?

Don't cry.
Shannon will be back after work
Would you like a magazine?

In hindsight, I realize that this is when Mom stopped reading magazines. She'd given up books in the past year, but still read newspapers voraciously and loved magazines. After this time at rehab, she didn't look at magazines again.

I put the flowers in your room
Can we check your blood pressure?
I need to GET your weight

Don't stand--
use the wheelchair

Talk to me
sitting

Sit Down

It's for your hip pain!
PAIN

Pills are for your Pain!
Pain!
PAIN
meds

These are your pain medications!

Dear Mom,
    Take your pills!
    Love, Shannon

Somehow, this worked. Maybe it was my name on the note or my familiar handwriting. When the nurse had a problem with Mom and her pills, showing her the note helped move things along.

Dear Mom,
    Need to put panties on
    Shannon

The aides learn quickly. This note isn't in my handwriting but its point is clear.

Dear Mom,
Put your Panties ON

That wasn't from me either. You notice there's no signature.

Put them on!

No excuses now, no cajoling. The panties have to go on. I can only imagine the battles that happen while I'm at work and my brain fills in her snarky responses.

From the back end of the notebook is another set of notes, these in my handwriting. I hoped, at the time, that Mom could reassure herself when she got confused. My notes are longer, full sentences, far too complex I see now.

This is rehab. They will help you recuperate from hip surgery.
Your leg is sore because you had an operation for a broken hip.
The doctor put in 2 screws to fix it.
The bruises on your arm and hand are from the IV at the hospital.
You will go home soon--about 1 week. They are keeping your room for you.

Then, in the handwriting of an aide,

Don't walk
Use your wheel chair.
You are sitting in it.

Mom: Sometimes I don't know what part of my life I'm in.

Me: Neither do I.

Going to Court

November 2004

    I have an appointment to meet Mom at eight-thirty. We don't usually make appointments to see each other. "Sunday afternoon about four" is the most definite we get these days. We meet for dinner after I'm done with work, rotating among four or five restaurants we have come to like near her nursing home. But today is Tuesday and we are not going out for dinner. I'm holding a subpoena in my hand and I check it again: Harborview Hall, Room 113, Seattle. We're going to court.

    Mom has been recuperating from a broken hip at a rehabilitation nursing home in Federal Way for a couple of weeks. I'd moved some of her things to make the place more recognizable. On the bookshelf, there's a picture of Grandpa standing with his first car. A favorite teddy bear that made the trip from California more than a year ago sits on her bed. A small notebook the staff uses to communicate with her is nearby. She doesn't look at any of these too much. The notebook makes her furious. "Talk to me, damn it! I'm not a child!" She cannot hear what anyone says. The hearing aids seem useless these days.

    A big fluffy cat called Artesia hangs out in the unit. She knows when she's welcome and when it is time to leave. Mom keeps forgetting whether or not she likes the cat. Artesia doesn't seem to care. She gladly flops in any available lap.

    Mom can't seem to hold on to the information that she's recuperating from surgery. "What am I doing here?" she asks again and again. "Who had surgery?" Although I visit her every day, she needs the litany of the events recited to her each time. My visits get shorter.

    Then things begin to happen. Mom refuses to cooperate with physical therapy. She spits out her pills. On the phone, I talk with the social worker. She says Mom threw a notebook at someone this morning. She is yelling, angry, furious, beyond words. "She's not doing well," the social worker says.

"She still hasn't adjusted from her trip to the hospital," I say, trying to figure out what might convince Mom to change her behavior. Reasoning with her isn't working. The social worker and I hammer out some strategies. Maybe I could be there when she gets her pills. Maybe we could hide the pills in her food. The social worker is concerned about the level of violence Mom shows. It's escalating. Mom was always prolific and creative at swearing, but throwing things doesn't bode well.

On the doctor's recommendation, Mom goes to a psychiatric ward. To get her meds adjusted, I am told. She is not happy. She is in a room with another patient. Mom doesn't tolerate roommates and she lets everyone know about it. She has to go through the Alzheimer's test again. "What year is it?"

"Who cares? I haven't cared since I retired."

"Who is the President?"

"That damn Bushie."

"What county is this?" I'm stumped by this one. Over the course of the last few weeks, we have been in Thurston, Pierce, and King Counties. Where are we now?

Mom's there at the psych ward for a week while they adjust the meds. I visit almost every day. She throws me out of her room, so I sit on the bench across from the nurse's station until she decides to come out and be social. I talk to other people on the bench. More than a few times, I think I'm talking to someone's family, only to discover that I'm talking to a patient. I wonder if people think I'm a patient. I haven't started throwing anything. Yet.

Now there is this summons for court. I won't have to do the transport. The hospital will take care of getting Mom there. I'm relieved. No telling what the ride in the car might be like with her so disconnected from reality.

The courtroom is in Harborview Hospital, the well-known trauma center for this side of the state. Injured people get flown in by helicopter. The care is first class. Buses come and go all day long outside, many of them filled with people coming for their mental health medications. I wait my turn. Only one case at a time gets heard in the courtroom. I look at the people around me and wonder, "Who is the family? Who is the patient?" It isn't always obvious.

It's a simple hearing. Just Mom and the judge and some paperwork requesting that Mom be required to stay another week at the psych ward.

When my name is called, I go to the courtroom. It looks like any good TV show set, but not as big as the ones on "Law and Order." Maybe twenty people could fit in here. Mom's not here yet. The judge shuffles paper and looks at her watch. Then the door opens and my mother sails in. She is on a gurney, sitting like a pageant princess. She's wearing a hospital gown and a blanket that doesn't cover her all the way. She's not wearing her glasses. The judge looks at her. This is not an unusual sight in this courtroom, I'm guessing.

The judge speaks. "Can you tell me your name?"

Mom shoots back, "Who wants to know?"

The judge licks her lips.

"Go ahead, lady." I roll my eyes and mutter, "You started it." And though I am sure I didn't say it out loud, the judge looks at me.

"Family?" she asks.

I raise my hand. "Daughter, your Honor" and we proceed.

Court concludes with an order that Mom return to the geropsych ward for another week. And then another. Three weeks all told and then she goes home to Olympia.

Chocolate Tacos

I hold up a dinner mint, one of Mom's favorites. "I brought you some chocolate."

"What?"

"Chocolate."

"Taco?"

I laugh. "No. Choc-o-late." I pronounce the word carefully.

"Taco," she says matter-of-factly.

"Chocolate," I say, matching her tone.

She frets. "I'm not getting what you're saying." I pop the candy into her mouth. She chews with attention. "It's good. I don't know what it is, but it's good." She turns away from me. "Can I see you?" she frets.

I tap her on the arm and wait until she turns toward me. Then I wave. "Here I am."

"What is it?" She is panicked.

"You wanted to see me. I'm right here." She shakes her head. It isn't the answer she needs.

Unfamiliar Territory

Spring 2005

Last week I got a call from a nurse at Mom's place. "Your mother pushed one of the staff." During the week, I talked with the mental health specialist who wanted to get Mom in to see a psychiatrist.

"Make the appointment. I'll get her there."

On Sunday night when I got home from work, there was a message, from another nurse. In front of several staff, Mom had pushed another resident, who fell into a woman who was in a wheelchair. The woman in the wheelchair had been thrown to the floor. The staff called 911. The wheelchair resident went out to the hospital in an ambulance. Just a precaution, I was told. The nurse asked about the appointment with the psychiatrist. "I haven't heard anything from the mental health specialist since last week," I said.

Five minutes later, my mother called. "There's been an incident," she announced. "You'll be hearing about it." We talked for a while. I told her that she would be going to see the doctor soon, that the pushing incidents were not like her. She was very confused. After years of working on picket lines with the farm workers, she is very committed to non-violence and can't imagine that she would shove or hit someone.

Monday afternoon, another call. They want to get Mom admitted to a psych ward that specializes in geriatric cases. Could I please come over?

I stopped at a store to find something to pack some clothes into. I had to make do with a huge "Happy Birthday!" gift bag.

I found Mom reading a newspaper in the TV room. Everyone else was out in the common area having a sing-along. She was surprised to see me. I told her we were going to see the doctor, that she'd be staying for a few days for an evaluation, and then she'd be returning here. We went to her room to pack and were out the door in half an hour.

She kept circling around the idea that she was being evicted and yelled at me when I didn't know how long the evaluation would last. She cried. She said, "I take my medicine every day. What is wrong?"

We stopped for dinner at one of our favorite places in Tacoma, and then went on to the hospital, another 25 minutes away.

They were ready for us with a big stack of papers that had to be signed. Mom was nasty to the nurse working with us, telling her she'd "rather talk to a MAN." We worked our way through the stack. The nurse said what each form was for, then Mom would be disgusted because she couldn't hear, or couldn't understand, what the nurse was saying, and then I'd translate it all. Then she'd sign and we'd go on to the next one. It took a long time.

Then it was time to check out her room. Her bed was by the window. She took one look at the bed near the door with a teddy bear at the pillow and threw a fit. She did not want a roommate.

Another nurse arrived with more papers to fill out. There was a brief physical exam, with Mom batting away the nurse's hand when she tried to check the hearing aids. Then there was more paperwork, again the list of questions for Alzheimer's. I could recite these in my sleep. Who is the president of the United States? ("that fool Bushie!") What season is it? What month? What day of the week? She got all those right. But "spell WORLD backwards" was just beyond her now. We gave it up. They'd try again in the morning when she wasn't so tired or upset.

She says it is time to die, that she never thought getting old would be like this. She imagined arthritis or losing energy, but not losing her mind. It is time to die.

She is tired, frightened, sad, bewildered.

Perhaps a thorough evaluation of her medications and her program will open the door to some new things: a fresh combination of meds, some suggestions for counseling or groups to participate in. She is a strong, bright woman and I think she's terrified by what she sees around her in other residents with Alzheimer's.

Mom Comes Home

Before I bring my mom home from the psych hospital on Monday, we stop for lunch at a local Denny's. She has a fruit bowl and a bagel with cream cheese. She hasn't had a bagel in a long time and she mentions that again and again. There are some food things we do for ourselves that go by the wayside when someone else cooks all the time.

Her hand often hesitates between the knife to spread the cream cheese and the fork for the fruit. More than once, she picks the wrong utensil for whatever she has in mind.

The drive to her place takes about 45 minutes and she naps in the car. When we get there, she wakes up. She smiles, pats my knee, and says how nice it was to be out for a drive. When we go inside, two of the staff members greet her, saying they'd missed her while she was gone. She looks as if she doesn't recognize them.

It is only later that I realize she doesn't remember being gone for three weeks.

Last night, I was going to bring her a "Welcome Home" balloon and flowers, but chose Valentine ones instead. She loves the foil-wrapped chocolate. I find her in the TV room, sitting close to the set so she can hear, without her hearing aids. She is sound asleep.

I wake her. "What time is it?" I tell her it's seven and she announces, "Then I can have all the chocolate I want. I've already eaten dinner!"

She's disoriented, very passive, sleepy. I worry about the slew of drugs she's on, including several antidepressants. We are getting an appointment with a psychiatrist very soon.

Two weeks ago, I would have said that she needed a facility with more structured activities and more residents who were still at her cognitive level. Today I am not so sure.

One thing I do know is that I am too close to it all at the moment.

> Mom: Do you have diphtheria?
>
> Me: No. I've been vaccinated.
>
> Mom: Oh, thank God!

The Hospital: Round Two

March 2005

Mom will have to be moved again. She has been at rehab since November, but this is an expensive place and Mom's finances can't handle it. Jacqui will do the research and I'll do the move, although Mom will go by ambulance, not in my car. I can't transport her in my car because she is no longer walking.

She hasn't stood up since mid-January. It was one thing to see her with a walker in the months after her hip surgery, but this is different. She is uncomfortable in the wheelchair and nothing makes it better. There are exercises she can do to improve her strength, but she won't do them on her own. If anyone assists her, she is dead weight, as if there is no connection between her brain and the muscles in her body.

The search for a new place gets refined. Now it is something as simple as finding a "female bed," not finding a good place for her to live. She is aware and not aware of her surroundings. One evening she said three sentences to me and then she fell asleep. She knows me less and less.

In the midst of this, Mom goes back to the hospital, this time with congestive heart failure and double pneumonia. For the first days, she has a high fever and isn't lucid at all. The pope is dying in Rome and the TV in Mom's room keeps running a retrospective of his life. Every time they use a bit of Gregorian chant, Mom makes the Sign of the Cross.

The woman in the bed next to her asks when her chicken soup will be delivered. "Half an hour? I'll be dead by then!" There is more Gregorian chant. Mom crosses herself.

She is vacant, stares into space or to a spot closer at hand. She doesn't register any movement near her. I know she will be gone one day, that it may be soon, or that she may continue like this for a long time. I hope I can stay with her in it, can simply be next to her when she needs me.

Mom's released from the hospital and "home" is now a nursing home close to my own neighborhood in Tacoma. It's an older building with great wide open hallways. There are no locks on the individual hallways, no special codes to get out the door. It's quite a walk from Mom's room to the front door. Maybe she won't make a run for it. She is worse every time she comes back from the hospital.

This time, the doctor says that Alzheimer's is affecting her swallowing and she isn't getting enough nutrition. We are going to have to think about a feeding tube in her stomach or letting nature take its course with hospice care on the horizon. In the meantime, her food will be pureed and we'll see if that works.

It took so little to move her this time: a small suitcase of clothes and some pictures. She has known me for ten minutes in the past two weeks.

A friend of Mom's came to visit. They've known each other since college days in the fifties. We found Mom in her wheelchair, slumped far over to the left. I tried to straighten her up and she hit me. "Leave me alone! Stop doing that!" She wore only a blouse and an adult diaper with a blanket across her knees. She has an awful rash at the top of her legs where the plastic of the underwear rubs against her.

She doesn't have her top teeth in. This is part of the battle with the new facility. I say she needs her teeth, even if she's eating shakes and pureed food. She needs them for talking, if nothing else. I'm told, "It really doesn't matter." But it does.

Mom's friend was shocked by the changes, though she stayed very calm. Mom never really woke up, never showed any recognition. Alice told me a number of stories about their travels in France, Mom not remembering to be somewhere, chatting in the bars with men—they in French, she in English, as if she understood them. She told me about their days on the Seattle University campus, all of that fifty years ago.

Now Mom has become one of "those" people in a nursing home. She fussed the first night about her ticket and whether or not she'd make her plane. But since then, nothing. She sleeps. Having a roommate doesn't bother her at all.

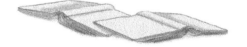

Rant from a Soapbox

Here is my soapbox. I have something to say—lots of somethings if I'm really honest about it. I've been avoiding paper and pen and people because I'm afraid if I get on the soapbox I won't ever get off.

First, my family. Do I need to break this down?

My mom has disappeared. In a few short months she has become unrecognizable. She remembered Mardi Gras in New Orleans but that was twenty years ago. An hour's conversation that won't be repeated. Since then, she stares through me, yells my name, doesn't know who I am. She has forgotten how to walk, doesn't recognize a tray of food, doesn't know what a newspaper is. I want to be furious but there is no one to yell at.

My brothers—when I cleaned out Mom's place last Monday, I found cards my brothers had written over the past eighteen months. "I love you! I'll see you soon!" One came for a visit last summer. We had lunch with Mom, she went to the bathroom, and when she came back, she had forgotten all about the lunch and complained that he'd only showed up to say hello and leave again.

Another brother sent cards and flowers but didn't show up. And another promised to come in December January February March. He hasn't come. "I love you! I'll see you soon!"

One of them complained Mom never answers her phone. Granted, maybe she wasn't in her room, but more likely she doesn't recognize the ring of a telephone anymore. One night I was visiting and checked her phone to see if it was plugged in. Then I dialed her number from my cell phone. Her phone rang, but there was no recognition in her face that anything needed her attention. "Your phone's ringing," I said, gesturing to it. She looked at me blankly and didn't move. I turned off the cell phone.

I cleaned out her room last week and it was all fairly simple: Goodwill, garbage, new place. Mom used to have the top half of a four-plex crammed with things she'd found at antique and second-hand stores. It took half a semi-truck to move her things from Santa Barbara and she complained for months about the shoddy service and how she was missing things. This time, I fit everything from her room into my car except the dresser and a fan. Half a dozen plastic sacks, a couple of boxes, and clothes on hangers. At the new place, she's down to three drawers and a closet. Hardly anything.

Doctors—let me yell at the doctors who kept her on a catheter for a month. What the hell was that all about? No wonder she doesn't want to walk. You've kept her in bed and in a wheelchair until she has forgotten she can walk.

And what about her walker? Where is it? Abandoned in physical therapy that she's not doing because no one explained that exercise will make her stronger and more able to do things.

She refused the cherry pie tonight because she doesn't eat other people's food. It took some time to convince her that the pie was hers. She said she was starving, she never gets anything to eat, but she didn't recognize the food in front of her. She loves ice cream when someone brings it and gets her meds in yogurt because she won't take them otherwise.

She used to love reading the newspaper and her magazines. No more. She doesn't know what a newspaper is and the magazines are confusing.

I've had a list for a week: change of address from the post office, notify the magazines of her new address, cancel the phone. I haven't done any of it because I know it means we have shifted to a new space.

My brothers—for all their promises to come see her—she won't know them when they come. She cannot name them. Their pictures are of someone else's children. She is not connected to them.

I am so angry that it has come to this. Mom doesn't get to spend her old age traveling, enjoying plays and symphonies and grandchildren. She doesn't get to be the slightly eccentric woman who had work and causes she loved. She doesn't get to enjoy good books and movies and funny stories.

She has become a terrified woman who sleeps most of the day in a wheelchair. No amount of cajoling or teasing or firm talk will change that. I do not like what I am witnessing. I do not know how to step back from it, or if I even should. I want to smash the soapbox and a few other things. I wish there were a way to smash the disease.

Losing or Letting Go?

Early summer 2005

Mom is living closer now, at a rehabilitation facility nearby in Tacoma, a place where they can deal with the Alzheimer's as well as her recuperation from the latest hospital stay. It seems to take more effort to see her now that she is living closer. Or maybe the problem is that she doesn't know me anymore and to see the extreme changes in her are really difficult.

Two years ago, we were out to lunch with relatives. A year ago, one of my brothers and his wife came for a visit. I used to be able to bring her books or magazines, or goodies to munch on. No more. She doesn't read anymore—she used to read three newspapers a day! Most of her food is pureed.

Each time she goes to the hospital, she loses so much. I can't do anything anymore. I can be there, talk with her, but she fades away or wants to know if we are related. The family doesn't seem to get it but what does "getting it" mean? This is simply how it is now.

When we moved Mom here, we didn't know how long she might be able to maintain. We hoped for two years. We got almost 18 months, and then the broken hip, the gero-psych ward, another fall, double pneumonia and congestive heart failure—and somewhere in there, she slipped away into a shadow world where she no longer makes a connection with the people around her.

What is she remembering? How much does she know right now? Does she comprehend what has changed? For a while last year, she would talk about how afraid she was. She would see the people around her and be frustrated by their lack of socializing. She didn't want to end up that way, but in the end, she has.

Is this what happens? That we become what we're most afraid of? I don't know if she was aware of the transitions. I was. I kept expecting her to come back to familiar territory, but she never did.

Each time she went to the hospital, she got a ticket to a new place and she has never been home again.

How will it all finish out? What will be the final episode? Will we know when it happens? I hope so. As deliberate as we have tried to be, I hope we know when the end is coming.

So much of the time since last October has been in adrenaline mode. Every time we settled, there was another crisis. Now it has been almost three months at this new place. A fall out of bed, a broken nose, bruises from her chair. No mad dash to the hospital. Things just are.

She has lost ground. She sleeps more, is more confused. Months ago, there were moments when she didn't know me, but only moments. Now it is reversed. She knows me for a second, if at all. I'm just someone who stops in to see her. "Are we related?" she asks. When I tell her she's my mother, she is puzzled. I wonder if she remembers having children at all. If she remembers me, she remembers a much younger me. Surely she's not old enough to have a daughter in her fifties.

Our conversations have moved to a new place. I rub small circles on her arm, just above her elbow. She seems to like that. She sleeps. I sit.

I am not who I was, the teller of funny stories about Mom's outbursts or strange responses. If I cannot tell those stories, who am I?

The Hearing Aid Saga

Dear Erin,

I'm glad it's Friday, but can I just say this? ARGHHHHHHH-HHH!

Mom's hearing aids are GONE. A couple of weeks ago I visited her midmorning. She was in the dining room, social time, not mealtime. She had no glasses on and no hearing aids. The occupational therapist came around to see if Mom could hear a little music box. When Mom didn't respond, I said, "She's practically deaf without her hearing aids." News to the therapist, I guess. I went to her room to track them down and got Mom set up.

A few days later, I was there after 6:30 p.m. Mom was in bed. Her hearing aids? Still in her ears. I took them out and left a note on the bulletin board. "Please take Marie's hearing aids OUT when she goes to bed." Leaving them in only causes the batteries to run down faster. The next time I saw her, no hearing aids. I asked the staff. No one knew anything. Just a great litany of "It's my first day." "I just got here." "I don't usually work here." We checked the meds cart. No luck. One of the workers said he'd pass the word on to the next shift. I wrote a new note for the bulletin board. "Marie's hearing aids are missing. Where are they?"

Later that week, still no hearing aids, but an answer was scrawled on the bottom of my note, "The son has them." Gee. Which of the four sons made a trip from California to snatch those hearing aids? And never called to have dinner? Really.

On Monday, I called to talk with the Resident Care Manager. "There's no son who could have taken those hearing aids. They all live in California. No one has been here for a visit for a long time." She promised to look into it and to have the social worker call me.

By Wednesday, I still hadn't heard from Margaret, the social worker. This phone call was the first she'd heard about the problem, and oh yes, she just started the job on Monday. I think I shall scream. She took *all the information, said she'd call me back, but if I didn't hear from her by Friday, please call again. She wasn't hopeful that they'd be found "after missing all this time." I insisted I had notified the staff as soon as I'd discovered those damn things missing.*

Friday. 4 p.m. Still no call from Margaret, so I called her. It was clear nothing had been done.

An hour later, she called back. She'd rounded up the staff and asked questions. One man thought he saw the hearing aids in Mom's ears a couple of days ago, but he isn't sure. They aren't in the laundry. Nor on the meds cart. But, Margaret says, "Maybe they were taken to the business office because they were dead."

I ground my teeth, bit my tongue, and seethed, "There are fresh batteries in her nightstand as well as a new package of them pinned to the bulletin board over her bed. Dead is no excuse."

The business office is closed until Monday.

The last time the hearing aids went missing, the nursing supervisor took them and put them in the (previous) social worker's office because "they didn't work." No one bothered to call to report the problem. Who knows how long Mom was without them that time. I ended up taking them over to the ear doctor's office. They swapped out the tubes and cleaned them up.

I told Margaret I have some big questions: like about that note that said, "The son has them." About procedures. About the care Mom is getting. Margaret suggests we might want to put Mom in another facility. Apparently she's too much trouble here.

More later. Film at 11.
Shannon

Weeks later, circumstances have changed. Mom has moved to another facility. Her hearing aids were finally located—at least maybe they were hers. I sent them off to the original maker in Santa Barbara who was able to trace the number on them and confirm they were indeed Mom's. The hearing aids were damaged, "sent through the wash," they said. Needless to say, Mom isn't the one who put them in the wash.

Who are You?

March 2006

    I sit down next to Mom and she looks at me with some interest. A visitor, someone has come to talk with her. "Who are you?"
    "I'm Shannon."
    "How did you get two Shannons in your family?"
    "There aren't. I'm the only one."
    "My daughter's name is Shannon."
    "I am your daughter." She looks confused, embarrassed. I have spotlighted the memory gap and she knows she falls short. Why do I do that? Why don't I just say, "I know you have a daughter named Shannon"?
    The mean part of me wants to yell. "Here I am! It's me! How can you forget me?" But there's no sense in it.

Linda's Game

May 2005

Mom has a black eye. "She fell out of bed and bumped her head." That is the first story we get. The doctor says her nose is broken. How did she fall out of bed? She doesn't move once she's in bed. And what did she hit her face on? No one seems to know. "It wasn't my shift" is a familiar refrain.

She was in good spirits last night and doesn't seem to be feeling any pain. She talked about the neighbors who are off traveling for a month. (Neighbors? What neighbors?) Her hearing aids are missing, but no one has walked off with the batteries yet. They are still pinned to the bulletin board.

We have yet to work out a consistent system for the nursing home to notify us when something has happened. Sometimes Geoff gets the call (he signs the checks); sometime it's me. It's hard to figure out who gets what information.

Mom's roommate, Linda, has a TV that is on all the time, turned up full volume with a parade of talk shows with outrageous guests who brawl and yell. If Linda's not in the room when I come to visit, I turn the TV off. Mom doesn't pay attention to it, but it's hard to talk to her over the noise.

Linda uses a wheelchair. She doesn't just use it to get from one place to another. There's an alarm that shrieks if she falls out of the chair. It also goes off if it is disconnected by a firm yank. Linda yanked that alarm again and again yesterday. People kept coming into the room to see if she was okay, to reattach the alarm, to scold her, to pay a bit of attention. She would grunt acknowledgement and when they left, she'd look around the room and pull on the cord again. It was almost comical, like watching a child—except that the alarm shrieks and almost drowns out the TV.

Mom is oblivious to it all. The noise doesn't even seem to register. She carries on a conversation, but I can't hear her over the noise. And she can't hear me. No hearing aids.

It Wasn't Supposed to Be Like This

MARIE: This wasn't supposed to be my life. When I retired, I expected to travel, eat new food, try new things, and see my grandchildren. I wanted to visit museums and send postcards from exotic places. I did go to Japan with my friend Alice. She complained that I was never where I was supposed to be on time. But a couple of years later, we went to France. That was a different trip.

We stayed at an apartment, tiny thing, with just enough hot water for the dishes or a shower, but not both. One night, we voted for showers, so Alice put a towel over the kitchen faucet to remind us not to do the dishes. But five minutes later, I was in the kitchen. "Alice? What's this towel doing on the faucet?"

We haven't talked to each other since that trip. I don't know what's wrong with her.

I don't see my grandchildren. I'm not sure I'd know them if I did see them. Sometimes I don't think I know my children at all. Have you met my daughter Shannon? Then there's Erin and (struggling) James and . . . When they were young, making noise and doing something they shouldn't, I'd just yell at them: Shannon, Erin, James. . . you know who you are! Quit doing that!

SHANNON: It wasn't supposed to be like this. This is the woman who lived and breathed books, magazines, newspapers. The bookshelves were always jammed and there were stacks of things to be read in her headboard. She loved politics and good arguments. She tried all sorts of restaurants, told great stories about enforcing civil rights laws.

In the last two years, she spent time in a mental health unit to adjust her meds, broke her hip, created such chaos in rehab that she was committed to a gero-psych ward, fell again, and went to the hospital with double pneumonia and heart failure. She talks to my father who has been dead more than 50 years. And my constant battle is with her damn hearing aids. Where are they this time??

Fixing Mom

Somewhere in me is the idea that Mom can be "fixed." If we figure out the right medications. If we can create a routine she likes. If she'd just see how she's acting and change.

But she can't be fixed. She just is. I have to get over being embarrassed, as if her behavior is proof of how badly I raised her. I think about that when I'm in the store and a child starts wailing. How the roles have reversed! She's living in a place where they know and understand the disease. I don't have to explain anything. As if explanations could prove anything.

But I do have to do something about the resentment. I resent having to keep track of her appointments as well as mine. I resent the responsibility of knowing her list of meds. I resent having to work my schedule around for two people. How do parents do this for their kids?

I'm often overwhelmed and resistant about dealing with Alzheimer's, except I never do deal with the disease. Instead, I deal with my mother who is more than a woman with the disease. She comes with all her history and all our shared history. I am a teenager all over again, trying to make sense of her inconsistencies and rages. How did she manage with six children? How did we not become just a mob to her?

In the old days, if someone was creating some kind of havoc, she'd start at the top of the list, "Shannon, Erin, James"—and then in frustration she'd say, "You know who you are! Stop doing that!" Even now, when she cannot name all six of us, I wonder if she ever could.

Of course she could. Surely she must have been able to. But it is hard to know. Those names are old; shouldn't they be the last to leave her memory?

Caught Spying

I have been spying on your life
    lifting bits and pieces
a few words here
    some gestures there.
I used to get whole scenes
    great dramas with an arc
        and climax
I could hardly write fast enough
    to get it all down.
"How's your mom?" people would ask
and I'd entertain them
    with another story.
They'd laugh
    or look shocked
    or say, "I don't know how you do it."
I didn't know either
    except that I kept spying
and stealing and writing.

The scenes got shorter
    the dialog disappeared
and my notes became invisible.
    There should be more stories
but there aren't.
There are only these lines
    and the memories shift shape.

I'm sorry for spying
    I just want to catch the story
        No—I want to catch you
before you fade into shadow
and become dust in sunlight.

Part III:
Now Where Are We?

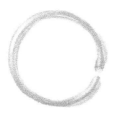

A Moving Interlude

September 2005

Tara calls me at work. She's a social worker at a nursing home that we checked out last week. We've been waiting to hear if they have a "female bed" that Mom could move into, but it was going to be a while.

Tara gets right to the point. "Did you know your mother was moved here yesterday?" This is confusing. Moved? We were just looking last week. She moved? How could she do that?

Tara says, "The senior shuttle pulled in around 11 yesterday. Your mom was on board."

"Did they tell you she was coming?"

"No." Stranger and stranger.

Fortunately, another resident was sent out to the hospital this morning, so there is a bed for Mom, at least temporarily. It takes a while to find out just what happened. The final report? Mom arrived in a wheelchair with a plastic garbage bag of some of her clothing and some of the things that had been on her wall. Was there paperwork? There was not. Was there a phone call from the other nursing home? No, not that either. So now what?

"Ask about her hearing aids," I say. "They were missing last time I checked."

Later I will find out that Mom was dressed and put in her wheelchair at 9:30, then parked outside the front door of the nursing home to wait for the shuttle. Someone told the driver where to take her, and that was it. The original plan had been for the new place to call the current one when a bed became available and then do the move. Paperwork arrived later in the afternoon, but we're lucky there's even a bed for her.

I make an appointment with the administrator of the rehab place. He wanted to know why I want to see him. I tell him we can start with their transferring Mom to a new facility without notifying the new place or the family. "Oh, we've already addressed that," he says.

"Not with me you haven't." Some of Mom's things didn't make the transfer, including a couple of teddy bears. They're looking in "dead storage" for those. The hearing aids didn't make it either.

Mom seems to take the move in stride. In fact, I don't even tell her that she has moved. Past moves have caused real distress and panic. Not this one. The staff works hard to engage her and keep her in the middle of activity.

The administrator at rehab claims it was all "a communication problem." No explanation for why they called no one about the move. I'm glad to have Mom out of there.

If My Mother Were in Charge

Well, there wouldn't be a roommate
    to start with,
but that's the least of it.

Mom's decorating has more style,
    let's face it.
She'd have coasters from Japan
    on the table
    and that print of the painter
    dangling from the Eiffel
    Tower hanging on the wall.
Her grand purple chair would be sitting
in the corner, with a splashy set of
    magazines
    decorating and travel mostly.
There would be some classy doorknobs
    in a crystal bowl,
promised for her next remodel.

Coffee mugs of several sizes
would hold her place in books
she'd picked up and set down.

Pictures of her kids,
stuck in grade school poses,
would line the bookshelves
and there would be twenty years
of letters stacked haphazardly
on the coffee table.

There would be a lovely throw over the
back of the settee—who has a settee

anymore? —a brilliant piece of fabric she
found in New Mexico and had to bring
home. A copy of the Elderhostel catalog
with new excursions for seniors would
be folded back, marked up, a dozen
possible trips in the future.

Next to the desk, where she used to write
out the household checks, would be an
indoor fountain. It's nice, she'd tell you
    but she never did figure out
    how to put it together.
Her purple slippers sit atop the week's
worth of newspapers from Santa Barbara
and San Francisco and New York.

There are only a few chocolate-covered
cherries in the box near the calla lily
 lamp stand.

But Mom didn't decorate this room.
There isn't much of her in it at all. A few
photos on the wall of people she doesn't
recognize anymore.

Cards to celebrate Easter, Mother's Day,
her birthday are tacked to the bulletin
board along with the reminder that she
must wear special socks.

Three teddy bears--one isn't hers—and
an orchid past its prime occupy the
nightstand.

Her roommate's half of the room spills
onto Mom's side. Stuffed animals,
scrapbooks, craft projects, a journal from
1999, they all hang from the curtain rod
and fall out of the bookcase.

Mom would have a fit
if she knew
if she could see and understand.

Her shoes have been lost. She probably
wears the largest shoes of anyone in the
nursing home; her black and white
athletic shoes are gone.

Gone too the deep dark red throw she
loved to touch. So much gone.

Today I brought her some new slippers.
They are shiny red with fake white fur
trim. She'd like them,
if she were in charge.

Talking at the People

Where are we-we-we-we-we...
    She struggles to finish the thought
We-we-we-we-we-we
    She waves a vague hand
    and then stares at a spot on the wall.

A few years ago
    She said, "There they come!"
    A crowd, she said, but couldn't say who.
    The dead?
        Her parents?
        Her husband?
I spot a man wearing a snazzy hat
    from the 30s. New York.
    He doesn't say anything — to me.
But she says, "Oh, it's you.
    I wondered where you'd gone to."
I try to interrupt.
    "Who is it?" She brushes me off and scolds.
    "You have your nerve."
He disappears into the moving crowd.

Later, in another place,
    "You were always such a disappointment."

"Adda adda adda adda," she barks it
    at the aide who comes to settle her into bed.

She's talking to the invisible people again
    I puzzle—she doesn't see me
    and she doesn't talk to me.

May 2008

Mom's Birthday 2006

"Happy birthday!" I say to the woman in Room 27. She is finishing her dinner, something with Italian tomato sauce. She turns her head slowly, her eyes almost refusing to make contact. "Happy birthday," I say again.

She wants to know, "Birthday? Whose birthday? Is it yours?"

"No, it's your birthday. I brought you a treat." I open the Dixie cup and put a spoon in the orange and white concoction. I put it in her hand, folding her fingers around the cold cup.

"My birthday? Well, that's a reason to celebrate! Here's to me!" She lifts the ice cream into the air and cheers. She digs into the cup. It is a warm day and the ice cream has already begun to melt. Almost half of it comes up with the spoon. She licks at it and tries to put it all in her mouth. "This is good," she smacks her lips. "How old am I anyway?"

"Seventy-six."

"Seventy-six?" She is appalled and amazed. Then she sings, "Seventy-six trombones led the big parade!" I laugh. She waves her spoon, conducting the band. "That's one of my favorite shows. I like musicals." A drop of orange falls from the spoon. She doesn't notice.

"You took us to see lots of musicals," I remind her. She'd bought season tickets for years to productions at the local junior college and we were treated to some of the best talent on the West Coast.

"King and I," she says.

I counter with "Guys and Dolls."

She offers, "Man of La Mancha."

"That was one of my favorites." I start to sing, "To dream the impossible dream, to fight the unbeatable foe…"

She looks at me as if I've lost my mind. "How do you know that song?"

"I saw the play when I was in high school. You took us to see it." She is puzzled. "Remember the long ladder that came down from the ceiling?" She doesn't.

She begins to fidget. The Dixie cup is empty but she is still scraping it. I take the cup and spoon from her and put them in the garbage. "Why are you here?" she asks.

"I came to celebrate your birthday."

"Birthday? I'm too old for birthdays. I don't care for them much."

"You used to make a big deal about birthdays, yours and everyone else's." She looks away. When she looks back, she is frowning. "What is it? What does it have to do with—with …" She struggles for words. "What does it have to do with circumstances?"

I am at a loss. It is time to go. If I stay any longer, she will start crying and make even less sense. She'll be agitated beyond her coping.

I give her a hug. "Good-bye, Mom. Happy birthday."

"Birthday? How old am I?

I wonder if she'll sing again if I tell her. I wait a beat and say, "Seventy-six."

She grunts. "Can't be. Not possible." She picks at her blanket and stares at the wall. She forgets me and I leave, but I am marching down the hall and I swear there are trombones somewhere nearby.

Mom: I haven't heard from your grandfather for a while. Is he all right?

Me: He's fine.

Mom: Is he still driving?

Me: No. He decided it was too much. A bit like going to church. He said he's done his pew time.

Mom: Does he live far away?

Me: It is a ways.

Mom: I suppose he sleeps a lot these days.

Me: I suppose so.

Grandpa's been dead for ten years, but he feels very close this day.

Theatre of the Absurd: Alzheimer's Style

It's summer 2007 when the phone rings.
May I speak to Mary Cain?
    No.
Why not? I must speak to Mary Cain.
    You can't. She is a patient in a nursing home.
May I have that number, please?
    No.
Why not? I must speak to her.
    She has Alzheimer's and doesn't speak at all.

May I speak to her husband?
    No.
Why not? I must speak to her husband.
    You can't.
Why not?
    He's dead.

Who are you? *He wants to know.*
    I'm her daughter.
Please fax me the papers that say you are authorized to speak for her.
    Who are you? *Now I want to know.*
Will you fax me the papers?
    No. Who are you?
I must have the papers.

*I hang up and dial *69. I get a phone number and I call back.*
    I say, May I speak to a supervisor?
Why do you wish to speak to my supervisor?
    I don't care if it is your supervisor. I want to speak to a supervisor.
Why do you wish to speak to a supervisor?

I want to speak to a supervisor.
We become dueling broken records. Finally,
One moment please.

This is David. I am the supervisor. What do you need?
"David" sounds very much like the man I first talked to.
David. What's the name of your company?
Why do you need to know?
Someone from your office called my home and wanted to speak to my mother.
Yes?

He would not identify the company or say why he was calling.
Yes?
I want to know why you are calling my house.
Please give me your phone number.
I do.
Then he tells me he works for a collection agency and says,

May I speak to Mary Cain?
No.
Why not? I must speak to Mary Cain.
You can't. She is a patient in a nursing home.
May I have that number, please?
No.
Why not? I must speak to her.
She has Alzheimer's and doesn't speak at all.

May I speak to her husband?
No.
Why not? I must speak to her husband.
You can't.
Why not?
He's dead.

Who are you? *he wants to know.*
I'm her daughter.
Please fax me the papers that say you are authorized to speak for her.
No. What is your business with her?
Will you fax me the papers?
No. May I speak to your supervisor?
He ignores me. I must have the papers.
I am silent.

I cannot give you any information without your paperwork.

We are trying to collect on five bills from an ambulance company.

Mom hasn't been in an ambulance for several years. Turns out the ambulance company has been sending bills to a place she lived more than three years ago.

I ask, Do you have the name of the power of attorney on your paper work?
Yes.
What name do you have?
I cannot tell you that information.
Do you have a phone number for that person?
I cannot tell you that information.
Never mind that the power of attorney has been listed on the paperwork for several years now. Two can play this game.
Call the number on your paperwork, *I say.* Thank you for your time. *I hang up.*

Geoff and Jacqui are on a trip for three weeks but I cannot give that information.
Good luck getting hold of them.

Making Plans

MARIE: Let's go out to dinner soon.

SHANNON: Okay. Tomorrow?

MARIE: That's good. I want Mexican food.

SHANNON: Sounds good. *(turns to leave and meets nurse)*

NURSE: What time are you picking her up tomorrow?

SHANNON: I'm not. I can't maneuver her into my car anymore.

NURSE: But you just told her you were …

SHANNON: And she won't remember the minute I'm out the door. Why upset her by telling her she can't go?

Words and More Words

Words are different altogether. Words I know and understand, like people. But the words that make up this story aren't the easy ones. They don't roll off the tongue without much thought. Instead, I must hunt them down, size them up, turn them this way and that, jam them into spaces and see if maybe, this time, the fit will be different. Even a few words and I am stymied. Do they fit this way? That way? Do they mean anything at all the way I have put them together? I close my eyes in the darkness, wanting the dark I can control rather than the one I cannot. I will not worry myself with how these words are strung together.

Mom used to reach for words, flapping her hand in my direction until she said, "You know what I mean." I usually did. I'd slip the word in, trying not to be obvious. Too many times I finished her sentences, talked over her unspoken thoughts, instead of letting her use the part of her brain that was becoming arthritic. Much of this was a pattern from the past. Mom and I had a long history of conversations on the phone over the years. For all the hours we talked, it was easy to fill in the blanks. When Alzheimer's asserted itself, we carried on as usual, not really noticing when the blanks got longer, the struggle for words more intense.

For a very long time, Mom's verbal skills were still good. She might make some comments out of the blue, but it was conversation and easy to get her on track. The last few years, the experience has slowly become different. At first, she'd try to find a word and pull a like-sounding syllable out of her storehouse. That usually gave her conversation partner a clue to fill in the blank and she'd pick right up and continue. The workers at the care facilities were adept at the game.

Later, her speech became half words, sometimes sounding like speech, with emphasis in the right places. It was tempting to respond in kind, speaking in tongues. I tried that early on. She looked at me as if I had sprouted a third ear in the middle of my forehead. She gave me The Look. I didn't do it again. It was disrespectful, I knew, and she'd give me a pile of grief about it the next time I dared try.

Much later, almost without noticing, she spoke in strings of syllables. There was no relation to the conversation. Harder still, she didn't seem to notice that she'd spouted gibberish. Where the syllables had once been the intrusion, now real meaningful words interrupted the train of thought. I jumped on the familiar words, tried to respond to those, but too quickly there was nothing left to respond to.

> Mom may be getting a new roommate.
>
> There's a woman who grinds her teeth and drives people crazy with the noise.
>
> Mom is deaf.
>
> Sounds like a perfect fit.

Attempted Conversation

I don't know if you ever told me
    my first word.
    Maybe you wrote it down
        in the baby book that has
    gone missing
    like so much else.
But knowing you
and your love of words
    and hearing echoes of you
    trying on words with each child
    all six of us
whatever the first word was
    you cheered
    you repeated it
    you bragged to anyone who would listen.
I'm sure you wrote it down.

Now after all this time
    libraries full of words between us
    strong lines that cross oceans and landscapes
    there are some signposts
        but most of the words are gone.

How can I write down your last word
    if you haven't said it yet?

November 2011

I Want to Be Here

April 2007

    I pull into the parking lot of the nursing home and shut off the engine. I sit there, looking at the other cars in the lot, trying to guess how many other people are visiting today. I don't want to be here. I have to be here. How could I not want to be here?

    I listened to a brief interview with Olympia Dukakis on the radio the other day. She went to see her mother one day and her mother, who hadn't known her for two years, said, "Oh Olympia, I've been looking all over for you!" They talked for twenty minutes and then her mother was gone again.

    I wish for moments like that. I can't even remember the last time my mother knew me and talked to me. A couple of months ago, I had a nice chat with her in the hallway. When I was getting ready to leave, she asked, "Who's coming next?"

    I told her, "Shannon's coming."

    "Shannon? My daughter?" She lit up with such anticipation and I didn't know what to say or feel. She remembers me but she doesn't know me. I wonder if this is payback for all the times I rolled my eyes behind her back.

    These days, if she's awake, she is focused elsewhere. I bring a chocolate bar with Paul Newman's face on it, guaranteed quality. She likes chocolate. I break off a small piece and give it to her. She closes her eyes and savors it. She can make a piece of chocolate last longer than anyone I know. She smacks her lips finally and stares into the distance again.

    She fiddles with her shirt, trying to pull it up over her arms. "Are you cold?" I ask but she doesn't answer. I go to find a blanket.

    There was a lady in the hall who has found a new mantra: "Help, help, help, help." She sounds familiar, but she's not the woman from that other facility who would walk the halls asking for help. This is an older woman and her chant is slightly off the beat of an emergency electronic beep. They never quite coincide. Both of them are trying to summon aid. It's Saturday, the staff is short-handed, no one comes. When the beeper is silent for a moment, I notice the silence and then the beeper resumes. Same person asking for help? Someone new? I don't know.

Mom likes the blanket. She's grateful for the warmth. I give her another piece of chocolate and absently rub her arm. "I miss you, Mom."

She looks at me, her eyes bright. "That feels so good." She's talking about the blanket. Or the chocolate. Or my rubbing her arm.

There's a bulletin board on the wall labeled "In Memoriam." It is full of obituaries, pictures and words about people who came through this nursing home and have gone on. I wonder if anyone notices while they're eating dinner. What a grim reminder. "Eat here and die."

The place smells today. Usually the smell of bleach is a subtle undertone in the air, but not today. Today the air is pungent with the smell of bodies and their cast-offs. If I stay long enough, I don't notice so much, but if I have to move from one room to another, the smell comes slamming into me.

I don't want to be here. I have to be here. How could I not want to be here?

Lost Connections

July 2009

I think we have reached the final stage in the progression of Alzheimer's. Again. After more than ten years of dealing with the disease, I don't know how I get fooled every time, but I do. When Mom fixated on being evicted, I thought, "Sheesh. Will it be like this forever?" It wasn't.

We would drive past an intersection and see someone waiting to cross the street, and Mom would say, "That woman is always there." No amount of discussion or comment would convince her otherwise. Will she always say this?

We went out for Sunday dinner and she complained that she never ate anything good at the assisted living place. But when I dropped her off afterwards, she didn't say good-bye, only "I can't wait to see what's for dinner tonight." Will this always be the way?

It was confusing. Maddening. Crazy-making. As we went along, I learned, learned to stay in the moment, to respond only to what needed a response, to not constantly correct her version of reality. My need to be right was seriously challenged. It was a discipline I didn't know I needed.

Ours was a noisy, vocal family when I was growing up. The sixties were challenging times. Local politics in small town California were just as fascinating as national politics. Discussions about teachers' union policies and strategies were not just for formal meetings. The talk spilled over into parties at the house. Their friends were as opinionated and vocal as my parents on all sorts of issues. To varying degrees, we kids read the papers, watched the news, tossed in our own thoughts. Our parents encouraged us to think through our positions. They played devil's advocate or suggested another perspective in another resource. Answers were never easy to come by. Good answers took hard work.

These days, there are no great raging discussions. Mom, who argued "Health care for everyone!" back in her high school class in the forties, would have loved the debates going on in Congress this summer. So what that it has taken sixty years for the rest of the country to catch up with her? She would be analyzing all the arguments and sending letters to Washington D.C., if she could. She would be on the phone to a few choice representatives and then she'd call me to tell me the latest.

When I sit with her now, she looks somewhere beyond me, her eyes not seeing much, just focused away from me. I hold her hand. I stroke her arm. I say her name. Nothing turns her gaze toward me. Inside me is a small child saying, "Mama, Mama, Mama," sure that if I just say it enough, or with the right inflection, she will turn and see me. Those moments are gone. We have slipped into this new place. I never thought we would be here. I had gotten used to her not knowing me, but for a long time, I could engage her in conversation. She might ask me if I knew her daughter, Shannon. "I hear good things about her," I would joke. She would tell me about Shannon's work at the prison and I'd say, "Must be very interesting work." Maybe I wasn't Shannon for the moment, but we could talk about her. We could talk.

We cannot talk now. Nor is there eye contact anymore. I look at her. She looks somewhere else, beyond me, beyond this time, beyond this place. I wonder what she sees. I wonder who is catching her eye now. Is it someone from the past? Is it a crowd of loved ones she recognizes? Or is it nothing? I don't know.

I mourn the loss of the crazy-making conversations when she'd talk about the "old biddies" at the other dining room table. I miss her weird stories about someone coming into her room and peeing into the wastebasket. I miss her looking at me and knowing who I am, telling me that my eyes look like my father's. The connection we shared with a look has gone, surrendered to Alzheimer's. I didn't know this was part of the price to be paid.

It's About the Teeth—Again!

February 2010

The day I visit, Mom's in the front TV room with half a dozen other residents. A lady with an IV attached to her arm asks me for help. But with what? She cannot say. It's warm outside, more like late April than late February, but it has been a strange winter. The daffodils do not bloom; they pop. The TV is locked on an infomercial for an exercise chair guaranteed to tone the abs. I look at the group in their wheelchairs. Doesn't anyone check what's on the TV?

Mom reclines in her wheelchair. It's slanted at the approved angle to prevent choking, or so they tell me. I think it's to stop any drool. Asleep, her arms are wrapped up in her shirt and her belly is bare. She tends to chill and no one remembers to leave her a lap blanket, so she's often exposing herself like this. I'm grateful she is so unaware, and then I'm angry. Dignity is not a complicated issue.

I've brought her chocolate, quality stuff I find at a discount and liquidation store filled with huge jars of salsa and boxes of mac-and-cheese dented from too rough handling. Mom would appreciate the store, and not just because she had a good eye for a bargain. There are treasures to be found on every shelf, if you can make it past the cheap bleach and the umpteen varieties of Rice-a-Roni. Artichoke hearts. Italian Wedding Soup. Orange and red peppers, two for a dollar. Spaghetti squash. It's never the same, although the good chocolate has its own shelf, and once I discovered it, I've made a habit of stopping by every week. I look like a crazed woman when I load up the basket.

I used to explain. "It's for my mom at the nursing home." The clerk would eye my well-fed self and smile. Nicely. I don't explain anymore.

In the TV room, the man sitting on the couch near the window has one leg tucked under him. He's wearing shiny green pants and drawing pictures in the air. He spots the bag of chocolate. "Bring that right over here, ducky. She won't be wanting any of that." I wave at him and smile.

Judy pulls up in her chair, hands curled with arthritis. "Going to share some of that, lady? I likes me some candy."

I open the bag and then the bright wrapper and offer her a piece. Judy opens her mouth wide and then clamps it shut. She closes her eyes and says nothing more.

I take a piece to the man on the couch. He winks, asks for a second, and I oblige.

I open another wrapper; this one has Mom's name on it. I rub her arm, trying to wake her. She turns her head to one side and I put the chocolate to her lips. "Hey, Mom, I brought chocolate." Not quite awake, she eats the candy anyway. She smacks her lips. "Oh, that's gooood." I'm delighted. I haven't heard a full sentence out of her in months. No full words either. I give her another piece. She takes her time.

I look at her face with its odd shrunken quality. She is wearing only her bottom dentures and the top half of her mouth collapses in on itself. She looks much older than she really is, until I remember she'll be eighty next summer. Still, if she had all her teeth in her mouth, she'd look different.

Mom gave up wearing top dentures more than two years ago. Too much of a bother, she told the aides. Her food has been blended and strained for so long, apart from the bits of candy she gets, there's really no need to chew. But the look of her face makes me think of the hearing aids she stopped wearing. And the glasses she decided she no longer needed. All that happened after she gave up walking and took up the wheelchair. I don't like the taste of all this in my mouth. Salt gathers at the back of my throat.

One more piece of chocolate. Mom is falling asleep. She hasn't said anything more, hasn't looked at me. Other residents are moving to the dining room. I take the bag of candy to her room to put it in the nightstand. The evening shift finds the chocolate useful as a bribe when Mom gives them a hard time.

I pull open the top drawer. Good thing I decided to come today because the candy supply is gone. Knowing the staff also enjoys the good stuff, I try to keep the supply fresh. In the corner of the drawer is a small, plastic-covered cup. There are teeth inside. I count them and then I head out to the nurses' station. I wait until the administrator has a minute for me.

I tell her I'm Marie's daughter and, "Could you have someone check on the teeth in Mom's room? There are more teeth in her nightstand than she could ever fit in her mouth."

The woman laughs with me, then raises her voice, "Search! Someone's missing their teeth!"

Guilt

Summer 2009

These days, I visit my mother about twice a month. I feel guilty about that at least 17 days a month. I should visit more often. I imagine the staff talks about me when I leave. "She almost never comes, never stays long." It is a deliberate decision to go to see Mom, every time. She doesn't live far from me, in the south end of town, right on my way to and from work. But I get in the car and I'm headed somewhere, or on my way home from work, and I look at my watch. Is it meal time? Do I want to go in during meal time? Mom is at a table by the window with two other people, people who can talk and sometimes feed themselves. Mom does neither.

There is a certain rhythm to meal time. Every person has a place at a particular table. I remember when Mom first moved to the assisted living place in Olympia. She used to complain about how snobby the other residents were. They never talked to her, never joined her at her table, and always seemed to make sure she knew she wasn't welcome at theirs. She didn't understand the concept of assigned seating. In Santa Barbara, meals were served cafeteria style and people sat where they wanted. There were those who had their set places, and God help you if you sat in someone's cherished spot, but a core of folks were relatively easy about who they sat with. I was amused one day to see Mom being uncivil to a woman who had recently moved in. After the woman turned to find another seat, Mom leaned across the table to one of her regular companions and said, "I can't stand her. She has nothing pleasant to say about anyone. Besides, what makes her think she can sit at our table?"

Mom had her own rituals for meals. Newspaper in hand, she'd drink several cups of coffee over the course of an hour or so. She'd read some bits of articles out loud to her companions and provide a running commentary, whether anyone was interested or not. Usually someone was. There was always some lively discussion.

The table here is smaller, room for four, but there are only three. The window takes up the fourth side. An aide on a rolling stool moves between this table and the one next to it. She positions napkins, puts silverware into unyielding hands, guides the milk glass to an uncertain mouth. She must feed one person at each table and so begins a dance of spoons and cups, first at this table, then at the other. Mom is mostly not interested in her food. If there's a spoonful at her lips, she'll eat. If there's not, she just sits.

When I come into this scene, I co-opt the stool and sit at my mother's table. I chat with the woman who can still talk. She tells me about her grandchildren or what she worked on that day. I tell her about my mother. "You look like her," someone will notice. I say, "There was a time when you couldn't tell us apart on the phone." I keep an eye on what food Mom seems to like best this day. It has all been run through a processor and looks like Glop, the infamous food we used to eat in college when we threw together the rice, vegetables, and whatever other leftovers we could find in the refrigerator. We used to joke about it being a multi-day meal. It was like thick stew the first day and could be fried by the third. Only college kids would eat it, but here it is, in the nursing home. Mom can't see it, so she doesn't protest.

I save the dessert for last. Most of the time I bring good dark chocolate. It's a good addition to the pudding that may show up. She likes the butterscotch pudding, is partial to the tapioca, and curls her lip when it's chocolate pudding. She always likes the chocolate I bring. I stroke her arm or pat her back. There's no use telling her who I am or trying to engage her in conversation. Sometimes she will start a sentence that collapses into repeated syllables. It almost makes sense. If I had the gift of interpretation of tongues, maybe we'd get somewhere. But that hasn't happened for a very long time. The lady across the table seems to appreciate my attempts to talk with her and when dinner is over, I give her a big smile and tell her how nice it was to spend some time with her.

If the room isn't too crammed with wheelchairs, I maneuver Mom's chair out of the dining room and back down the hallway to her room. We sometimes sit in the hallway, out of the traffic. I hold her hand and read poetry. She falls asleep in her chair. I pull the blanket up around her and leave.

I cannot put her to bed. There's a machine that lifts her out of the wheelchair and transfers her. Getting her ready for sleep is a two-person job and I don't have the requisite training. I tell her goodnight and leave.

I haven't been there very long, no more than half an hour. There is nothing to say. I get in my car and drive away. Maybe next time I'll stay longer. Maybe next time she'll say something I can respond to. Maybe next time she'll know who I am. I don't know if I can come back. I know I should. I have to. She's my mother. But the long stretch of not being known is getting to me. Every time I go, I have hope that we will return to a former plateau. We never do, but I still hope. I don't feel like the "good daughter" who is selfless and giving and puts her mother first. I am often fitting her into the rest of my life, shoehorning a moment. I know I don't have to stay long because she doesn't know how long I stay or if I come at all.

Calling Mom

29 April 2010

    I picked up the phone to call Mom today. I had something to tell her. Something about a new job prospect. I was going to talk out the pros and cons with her. I love my job and she thinks my job is fabulous and exciting, adjectives that I always gave to her jobs. She's a forward-thinking woman and never let herself be limited by traditional roles. When I was growing up that meant teacher, nurse, or secretary. She taught for a while, even showed up in one of my high school classes as a substitute, but left that to become a reporter at a newspaper. She was a stringer, paid by the story, rather than a hired reporter. She worked on those stories. She found unusual people and even better tales about what they'd been up to.

    I punched in her number on the phone and waited for the ring. On another phone, in a different decade, she was on speed-dial. I never thought about the number. It was on that third button from the top, left hand row. Punch that button and Mom was right there, usually saying, "I was just thinking of calling you" as soon as I said hello. We did that all the time. Some of that family telepathy, I think. I've never perfected it with my siblings, but Mom and I? We're experts.

    She didn't answer, of course. "The number you have dialed has been disconnected or is no longer in service. Please try your call again." I listen to the recording again and then I hang up. Of course she didn't answer. She doesn't have a phone anymore. Doesn't have conversations any more. As far as I know, I'm not her daughter anymore.

Another Birthday 2010

A few months ago, the youngest of the siblings sent out an email and said, "Mom's turning 80. Let's have a party!" My first instinct? "Hell no." It was selfishness on my part, not wanting to let other people into my experience of being with Mom who has changed so much.

Four years ago, Mom sang "Seventy-Six Trombones" when she found out it was her birthday. She was still talking then, still able to enjoy some messy ice cream and to talk about different musicals she'd seen over the years. Things are different now.

It has been six years since that youngest son has seen her. She was up and walking then. We had lunch together and she left to go to the bathroom. When she didn't come back, we went to find her at her room. When she opened the door, she welcomed us as if we'd just arrived. After a few minutes she said, "You've been here for a while, haven't you?" We had. "Have we had lunch already?" We had.

The oldest son hasn't seen Mom in fifteen years, at her father's funeral. He is anxious, unsettled, hasn't wanted to see her in this state, so unlike her old self. His wife finally prevailed upon him. "You have to see your mother," she said, "for your own good."

So we collected ourselves over the weekend and on Sunday at one, we showed up at Mom's nursing home. The dining room was full of residents and some visitors, and the very capable staff who each managed to supervise a table of four while feeding at least two.

Crispin ordered a chocolate cake with raspberry filling from a local bakery. We handed around pieces of cake to anyone whose stomach could manage it, including the guests in the room. Every aide got a piece, including a few who came in because they'd heard there was cake on the premises. There was still a quarter of the cake left at the end. We sent it to the staff break room, certain there was still enough to go around.

Pictures were taken with half a dozen cameras and phones, the family group mixing and melding into various configurations. We haven't taken pictures like this for a very long time. A copy of one of these will go on Mom's nightstand, along with one from her parents on their sixtieth wedding anniversary. The last good picture of Mom and the six siblings was taken in the '80s. It was mid-afternoon on a summer day and ended in what has come to be known as the Great Fig Throwing Event, definitely the stuff of family legends.

These new pictures capture us in our late forties and fifties, the same age as Mom was that summer afternoon. I know we didn't think then of where we might be when Mom was eighty, but here we are. We are still trying to make an occasion of things, still working at making a family unit. Maybe this won't be the stuff of legends, but we try.

Placeholder

I've buried you
    a couple of times
maybe not all the way
I haven't dug the grave
    but I confess to picking out
    the music
and wondering if we could
    afford the limo.

I've been methodical about it
    especially after those trips
        to the hospital
    those times you left a part
        of yourself behind.

You never really came home.
    Not all the way
Did you send someone to be
    your placeholder
        to remind me you're still here
        even when you're not
        not all the way?

After Words

It is the spring of 2012. It has been nine years since my mother moved from a retirement home in Santa Barbara to Washington. She lives in a nursing home only a few miles from where she grew up in South Tacoma. She will be eighty-two this summer. Her general health is good. Her medications are few. Her swallowing instincts are enough to allow her to eat regular food instead of having it all pureed. Non-vegetarian food sometimes slips in, but she only smacks her lips and will eat more. She spends most of her days sleeping, sometimes in her bed, more often in her wheelchair. She still loves chocolate in any form.

I can't point to the day when Mom didn't know me anymore. It happened slowly. She'd forget for a few seconds and then remember. It feels like a very long time ago now that we had any conversation that made some sense. When I spend time with her now, we sit together in silence. I hold her hand or rub her arm. Every now and then she will wake up enough to be aware of my presence but those moments are now weeks apart, almost months. The days of getting good stories out of her are unimaginable now. My stories about her became shorter over time and then lost their variety. "How's your mom?" people ask.

"The same," I say. "She sleeps."

"But she still knows you, right?"

No, she doesn't.

I'd like to think that somewhere in her is a memory of who I am, like she remembered Bob and the days they had together back in the fifties. But I can't be sure of that. After a certain point, you can't know. I hope she carries in her some memories of the rowdy household of kids, the people she worked with, the travels she took. But I can't know.

"How will you know when you're done with your book?" For a long time, I didn't know. Maybe when Mom died, when we'd had her funeral, and distributed what was left of her stuff. But that hasn't happened yet.

What it has come to is this: there are no more stories to tell.

I'm disappointed. I thought there would be funny stories all the way to the end. I was wrong. There were many funny things. Many exasperating things as well. These years have been a time of knowing my mom, one adult to another, and then marking the shift and almost the reverse. Who is the parent here?

Over the years, she found a reason to stop driving and to move from Santa Barbara. She stopped asking for good coffee and was satisfied with water thickened so she wouldn't choke. My mom found reasons to give up her watch, her glasses, her hearing aids, her upper teeth. She gave up her stories and memories and relinquished familiar names.

She gave up her fear and terror about the effects of Alzheimer's, let go of the paranoia of being evicted, and at some point, gave up the ferocious anger that gave her the energy to survive the first years of living in a care facility.

I remember a day in the hospital in the spring of 2005. She was unconscious, but as the news reported on John Paul II's last illness, punctuated by Gregorian chant, she blessed herself, as she had done as a girl, as she had taught her children, as she had stopped doing decades ago.

There are no more stories to tell. And I've been missing her for a very long time.

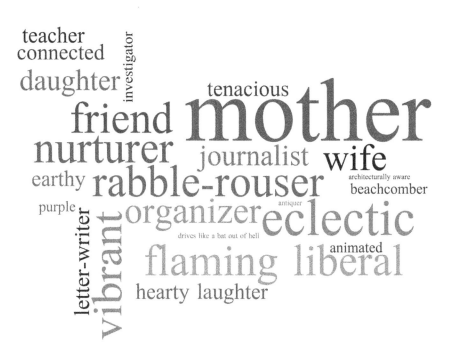

After Stories

An early morning phone call sends me to Mom's nursing home at eight. The caller says Mom is having some trouble; they'd found blood. It has been years since there's been any urgent call or something to worry about. I pull out my wooden stool from next to the night stand and sit down. Mom is sleeping. The head of the bed is raised far beyond its usual position. She is almost sitting up. Her breathing is rough, even with the help of oxygen.

An aide comes in to check on us. He gives me a few more details and says, "We're waiting for the doctor to come." Beyond that, no other news. He adjusts the oxygen tube and leaves. We sit together, me watching her, counting the spaces between breaths.

It is mid-November 2013, a bright Sunday morning. I hold her hand and start naming names. I begin with her first husband and my long-dead father, with my grandparents, with Mom's college friend who died suddenly in June, with Dawn and Sr. Una whose funerals happened in the last two weeks. I think of the long list of names remembered at my parish's All Souls Day prayer service and the wall of names listing the dead from wars in Afghanistan and Iraq. Lots of saints and friends to call upon, which reminds me to phone my friend Judy who will be on her way to Mass soon. I tell her Mom is very sick and ask her to put Mom's name on the prayer list at church. I pick up her hand again and watch her breathe.

Sunday morning in the nursing home has a different rhythm from the late afternoons when I usually come. It is busy with the ordinary shuffle to breakfast. A side door opens and closes for the smokers. Most of the residents and the staff are clustered near the dining room, half a hallway away from us.

Mom's roommate never leaves her bed. She's awake behind her curtain. The TV is on. Betty is very fond of golf. This is not golf she's watching now. Mom catches her breath. The play-by-play continues. Hushed voices explain the strategy. Silence. Then a cheer. Point scored! No. Not golf. It's a curling competition.

Mom's breathing gets quieter. Betty changes the channel. Cars race around the track while the crowd roars.

A volunteer comes in the room with a small dog. "I hear you might need some company," she says. I look at her. I look at the dog. Mom is not a fan of dogs. Neither am I. "Thanks, but no." The visitor notices that Mom is struggling a bit and takes a few minutes to dampen a cloth and put it around her neck. Mom sighs.

I talk with the aide again. He says that Mom's organs are failing. "She's dying?" It takes me a minute to understand. I thought this was just a blip on the screen, something solved with medication. Isn't the doctor coming? Mom's dying?

"We can transfer her to the hospital if you want."

"No. Thank you." The answer comes quickly. Mom has lived in this room for most of the eight years she has been here. This is home with all its sights and sounds and smells. An ambulance ride and admittance to the hospital where she would be placed on a bed in a sterile room, new people working with her? Mom has a "Do Not Resuscitate" order on file. What would the hospital be able to do? No. Thank you. We'll stay here. If Mom is dying, she will do it in this place, in this bed.

He nods. He knows the routine. He's had this kind of event on his shift many times. He promises to check back in.

It's after nine. I call my sister in Oregon, then my brothers in California. One makes plans to fly in the next day. No, I say, she's dying. She'll be gone. I call my Mass-going friend again with the update. My sister is on her way. I go back to Mom's room.

For the next hour, Betty switches among the channels: curling competition, racing cars, infomercial. Background noise of the strangest kind. Outside, the sun lays claim on the day and the traffic on Pacific Avenue is steady. Mom's breath catches every now and then. Her hand stays within mine. We wait.

Some blood trickles from her mouth and then some more. I get a towel to clean it from her chin and go to find the aide again.

When he checks on her, he nods. "Her organs are shutting down." He said that before but now it is more final.

Betty has found another competition: brides trying to find their perfect dresses. One wants to look like Grace Kelly; another is in love with Princess Diana, even had a talk with her that very morning. Mom would cackle at the absurdity. It's after ten. I think of the parish gathering for Mass at 10:30. The warmth of their prayers surrounds me.

Mom stops breathing.

Starts again.

I round up the long-dead relatives and the newly-dead friends. "She's almost there. Get ready." It's not hard to imagine Mom stepping into the party. The gaps between her breaths are longer. I don't count the spaces. The brides go on with their dress-hunting and I'm aware that I'm amused by taking note of them while I'm sitting here waiting for my mother to die. She would get it. She'd laugh. I know she would.

Just before 10:30, she doesn't breathe again. Ever. No matter how long I wait. No matter if I talk to her. No matter that I wish it, want it, pray for it. There is no more. She is gone. I hold her hand still. Nothing has changed except she is not breathing.

We stay like that for another ten minutes before I tell anyone.

At the nurses' station, I report that she has died. I call my sister, who is on her way from Portland. I call one of my brothers and ask him to tell the others. I call the funeral home.

Back in Mom's room, someone has lowered the bed so she is now lying down. Her face has been washed, the blankets pulled up. Some of the workers stop in to say goodbye.

When the man from the funeral home arrives, we meet across a table to fill out forms. I've dealt with this mortuary many times over the years, both for family and for work-related things, so our conversation is almost comical. I go back and forth between the grieving daughter and the church professional. We get the papers done.

My sister arrives with her grown sons, so together we go to Mom's room again, to spend some time with her. We escort her out to the hearse.

My friend Lynne arrives with empty tote bags. We clear out the closet and the night stand, pack up what we want to keep, set aside what can be donated, pull out what isn't Mom's but has ended up in her keeping. Betty gets what's left of the chocolate. Then I pick up the wooden stool that I brought in eight years before and we all go out to the parking lot. We're going to lunch.

On the first weekend in December, the family gathers. The memorial service is held at St. Leo Parish. Mom went to high school here. Grandpa was buried from here almost twenty years ago. Mom had given up on church, except for attending Unitarian churches that "have great potlucks." A wall hanging with pictures from her life stands behind the table where we place her ashes. Mardi Gras beads and a child's set of china made during the war years tumble out of a wooden box. We tell stories about her work with the farmworkers and how she took delight in nailing people who denied housing to persons of color. At the reception afterwards, two of her high school classmates confirm a story about a prank Mom and some friends pulled back in the '40s. A CD compiled by Judy plays songs that Mom loved, including selections from *Jacques Brel Is Alive and Well and Living in Paris* and *Save the Bones for Henry Jones*. It is a fine celebration. We take the box with her ashes when we leave.

A final dinner that night and then Sunday and Monday we go our separate ways.

After a few mix-ups and "what the hell" moments with the cemetery, Marie Cain is finally placed in a columbarium dedicated to St. Francis of Assisi, not far from her parents' crypts. It is outside, sheltered from the wind, exposed to the sun and rain. She's on the "bottom floor." The lady at the cemetery told me of a man who'd come in to make his arrangements and claimed the top row, corner niche. "I want to see who's coming around." Mom was never much interested in that. A place near the ground puts her close to kids and animals—and saves a few hundred dollars.

It's still a shock to remember that she is gone. There are reminders of her. Each of the siblings has a copy of the music CD and it is a staple in my car. The banner with the pictures of her life hangs in my living room. Every now and then that episode of brides choosing their gowns shows up on TV. I consider that a nudge from Mom. Her odd and silly chants come to mind when I least expect them. I'm sometimes tempted to one-up the swearing I hear with Mom's far more colorful examples. Most of all, I remember her in discussions about politics and in work that is about justice. It's a good legacy.

Here's to you, Marie Margaret Ultsch O'Donnell Cain.

Spring 2016

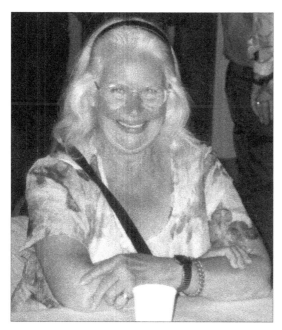

Marie Margaret Ultsch O'Donnell Cain

Some Words of Thanks

"Help me, help me, help me. Thank you, thank you, thank you." Writer Anne Lamott claims those are the only prayers a person needs. Or she did. Recently she amended the list to include "Wow." How fitting.

There are many people who have helped me over the years: family, friends, co-workers, fellow writers, people who made me laugh and those who made me cranky. To all of you, thank you. I'd list you by name, but find I have to pull a page from my mother's book and say, "You know who you are! Keep doing that!"

Thanks, Mom.

Wow.

CPSIA information can be obtained
at www.ICGtesting.com
Printed in the USA
FSHW011950190120
66275FS

9 780982 616048